LESLIE KENTON'S
COOK ENERGY

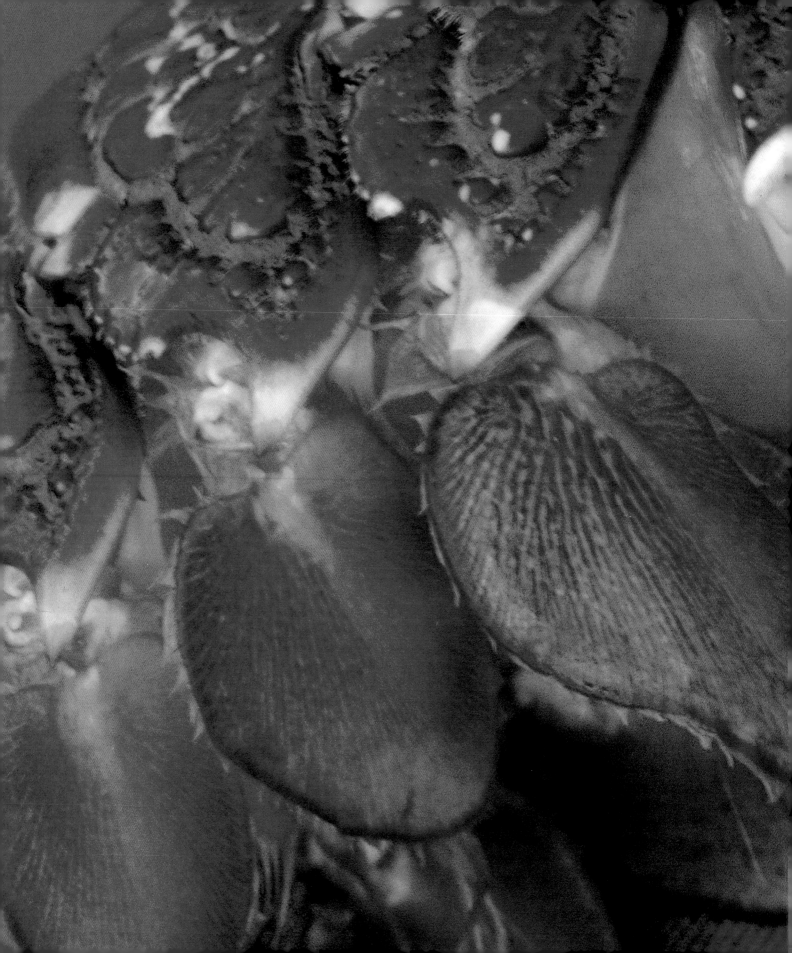

LESLIE KENTON'S
COOK ENERGY

Lean Feasts, Vitality Secrets and Power Foods
to Help You Live Longer, Look Younger, Feel Better

Photography by Leslie Kenton

TED SMART

This book is dedicated to my youngest son **AARON** whose creativity inspires me
whose laughter sustains me
whose clarity dazzles me
and who makes great
teppan yaki

This edition produced for The Book People Ltd, Hall Wood Avenue,
Haydock, St.Helens WA11 9UL

1 3 5 7 9 10 8 6 4 2

First published by Ebury Press,
Random House, 20 Vauxhall Bridge Road, London SW1V 2SA

Random House Australia (Pty) Limited
20 Alfred Street, Milsons Point, Sydney, New South Wales 2061, Australia

Random House New Zealand Limited
18 Poland Road, Glenfield, Auckland 10, New Zealand

Random House South Africa (Pty) Limited
Endulini, 5A Jubilee Road, Parktown 2193, South Africa

The Random House Group Limited Reg. No. 954009

www.randomhouse.co.uk

A CIP catalogue record for this book is available from the British Library.

Editor: Emma Callery
Designer: The Senate
Recipes prepared by: Shirley Bradstock
Styling by: Amanda Cooper Davies

Papers used by Ebury Press are natural, recyclable products made from wood grown in sustainable forests.

Printed and bound in Singapore by Tien Wah Press

AUTHOR'S NOTE

The information inside is in no way intended to be prescriptive, to replace medical advice, or to be a substitute for a good doctor or well-trained health-care practitioner – especially one knowledgeable in nutrition and natural healing. If you are ill or suspect you are ill it is important that you see a physician. If you have been taking prescription medication, don't change your diet drastically without consulting your doctor. Neither the publisher nor the author can accept responsibility for injuries or illness arising out of a failure by a reader to take medical advice. I want to make clear that I have no commercial interest in any product, treatment or organization mentioned in this book. I do, however, have a profound interest in helping myself and others to maximize their potential for positive health, awareness and creativity. For it is my belief that the more each one of us is able to re-establish harmony within ourselves and with our environment, the better equipped we will be to wrestle with the challenges now facing our planet.

CONTENTS

COME ALIVE

Put away your kitchen scales and forget the complex routines for preparing a béchamel sauce. Cook Energy breaks all the rules. For it is not rules that matter when preparing foods, it is a kind of passion for the foods themselves - a feeling reflected in our passion for the earth and for life itself. You see it in a small child as he enthusiastically devours a bowl of fresh strawberries drizzled with honey. It's good because it tastes good. Such passion, which is visual, visceral and sensuous, becomes the inspiration, which in food preparation leads you automatically to make certain choices. If two things look good together they taste good together.

YOU WOULDN'T PUT OCTOPUS AND CHICKEN IN THE
SAME DISH.

Open wide your kitchen window. Welcome the breezes of experiment, wit and spontaneity. Inside, you will find the traditional meal of roast meat and boiled Brussels sprouts topped off with a piece of sticky toffee pudding replaced by something far more hedonistic. Slivers of raw Pacific salmon, luscious garden-fresh salads with a slice or two of Russian black bread followed by a winter sorbet of cranberry and mint are what is on offer. These foods are lighter, richer in protein and full of texture, flavour and surprises. Most of the recipes are easy to prepare and all the foods they call for are chock full of the newly discovered nutraceuticals - natural plant and animal chemicals - to help you look good and feel great decade after decade. The real joy in eating fresh, light, protein-rich foods lies in their taste, their texture and the remarkable ability they have to bring excitement to a palate jaded by too many highly processed, unimaginatively seasoned or over-cooked dishes.

I love these recipes, first because they taste delicious, and second because together they make up a way of eating and living that supports the body and the highest levels of energy and well being. I look on food as a source of both delight and life-energy, which is passed on to us from the earth. I believe this energy needs to be preserved by not cooking food too much, by eating it fresh and by respecting its essential nature. Food eaten this way becomes a medium through which we build our own vitality - energy to protect the body from premature ageing and illness, to enhance good looks and to keep the mind clear. It is the life-energy present in abundance in fresh foods and the clean, simple protein from fish, game, organic meat and poultry that makes these foods irresistible and helps us to look and feel great.

WHAT IS COOK ENERGY?

A new approach to food preparation, Cook Energy is based on creative play, excitement, experimentation and sensuous enjoyment of fresh foods, which enhance health and looks in medically measurable ways. There are no 'sins' in a Cook Energy foodstyle. The very concept of 'sinful food' touted by slimming clubs and health fanatics is offensive to me. You don't choose a food because it is good for you. You choose a food because it is good.

Pick foods that excite, inspire and delight you. Cooking is a process of experimental and imaginative play. Never follow a recipe by rote. To me that would be boring – the kind of 'sheep' mentality that went out with the last century. The recipes in this book are in no way designed to be imprisoning. They are meant to be inspirational – to encourage you to explore the infinite possibilities of creating wonderful meals for all occasions with minimum effort and maximum fun.

In energy cookery it is not rules that matter. It is a kind of passion for the foods themselves, which is reflected in an affection for the earth and for all life. This passion leads you to make certain choices in food preparation. In fact, the passion itself becomes a kind of inspiration. If two things look good together they taste good together, and vice versa. You wouldn't put octopus and chicken in the same dish.

Fresh, organic foods untainted by chemicals – the sort of food your grandparents probably grew for themselves – form the raw materials of Cook Energy. Why? Because these foods are both the most delicious and the most life nurturing. Values in cooking and eating are making quantum leaps. Food now is lighter, richer in protein and full of texture, flavour and surprise.

In case you think you should eat lighter, fresher foods because they will keep you from having a heart attack or prevent inches from creeping up around your waistline, forget it. I think the word 'should' has far outlived its usefulness. Oh yes, it is true that Cook Energy foods will do all of these things. A diet rich in fresh vegetables does indeed help prevent cancer and other degenerative diseases. It even slows ageing. But the time when we were told to get plenty of protein or bran, to eat this and not eat that, just because it was good for us is over. The real joy in eating fresh, light, protein-rich foods lies in their taste, their texture, and the remarkable ability they have to bring new life and excitement to a palate that has become jaded by too many over-processed, or unimaginatively seasoned dishes.

START AT THE BEGINNING

Cooking starts at the shopping stage. It is when you are in the market surrounded by great mounds of lettuces, avocados, fresh peppers, parsley and squid that you get your inspiration. Never

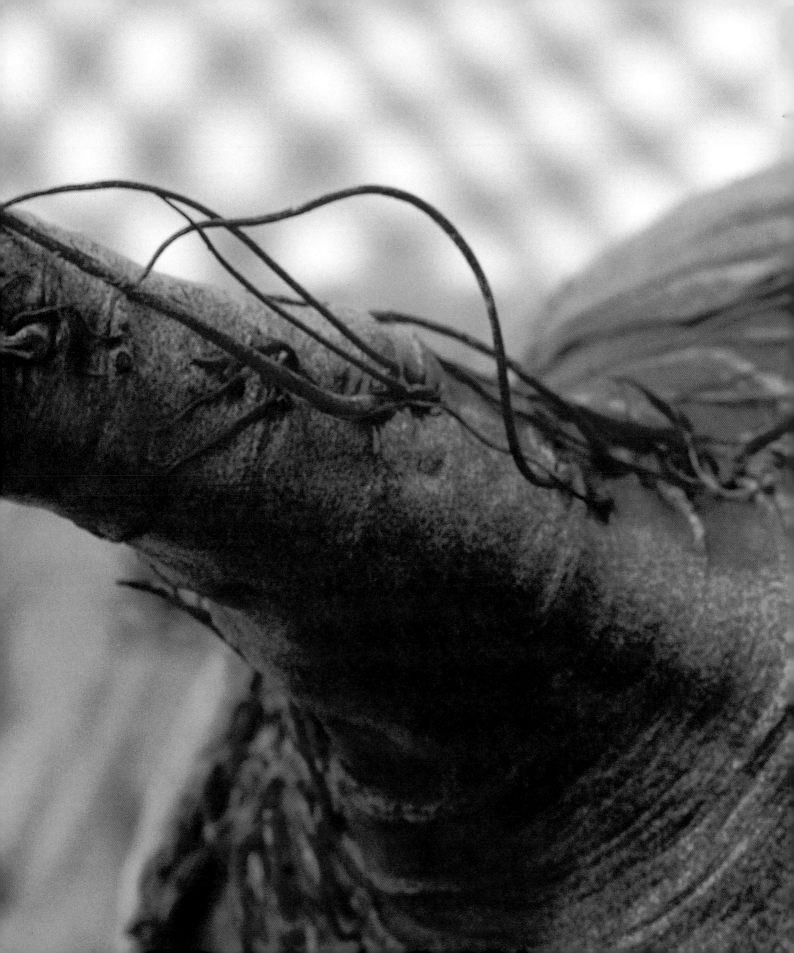

set out to buy food with too fixed an idea of what you intend to buy. Look for what is particularly cheap. Some of the very best dishes can be made from the commonest vegetables such as carrots, turnips and watercress. Often the cheapest fish is the most tasty – provided you know how to prepare it. You may come across something that, although you have not thought of it, is beautiful. It draws you to it. Buy it. Forget what you thought you were after. A good menu is created while you shop.

Why seek something that is not there or out of season? Fresh foods bought in season offer the highest complements of vitamins and minerals you can get. Even better, they are rich in phytonutrients – plant factors such as lycopene, co-enzyme Q10, and the remarkable flavonoids. These plant factors are so effective in enhancing health and good looks that if they are missing from your diet (as they are from the diet of all who rely on convenience foods) then you are quite simply missing out on vitality at the highest level. Let yourself be tempted by all the gorgeous vegetables and fruits you find. Make them the focus of your menu. Always seek temptation. To enjoy food fully, to celebrate the beauty of food, your senses need to be heightened.

BREAK THE RULES

In the realm of cooking a whole new ethos is being born. You don't need to have every ingredient to make a recipe work. I love coming into my kitchen and making a meal out of practically nothing – wilted spinach, whatever herbs I have in the garden, four eggs, an apple, half a carrot and a piece of fresh ginger. These recipes are great fun to prepare. Don't get hung up on measurements. Use them only as guidelines. Try a little more of something, a little less of something else. If you like the look of a recipe but don't have all the ingredients, then substitute. One of my sons, Jesse, once decided to make banana bread. The recipe called for nine ingredients but he had only five. Nevertheless he managed to toss them together, whip them up, and create what everyone in our family thought was the nicest 'Banana … err' that any of us had ever tasted.

QUICK START

Who, these days, has time for breakfast? Yet breakfast is the most important meal of the day. Not that you need to stuff yourself with food you don't want for energy. That is an old wives' tale. But everybody needs something first thing in the morning, whether it be a cup of good coffee, a glass of fresh vegetable juice or fruit juice, an apple, a fruit smoothie or some good old-fashioned porridge which is waiting for you when you wander sleepy-eyed into the kitchen.

There is a quick start breakfast that is just right for you. You may be someone who thrives on a sense of emptiness, in which case reach for a glass of fresh juice, which will let your body continue the process of inner cleansing that takes place each night clear through to lunch. You may crave something fresh and fruity but more substantial. Try a peach smoothie. If you are one of those people who never gain weight, no matter what you eat, you are better off going for an instant wholemeal porridge. Experiment. Find out what works best for you. Don't be afraid to change with the seasons either. The body and psyche are always evolving. Let how you eat evolve too.

LET BREAKFAST BE NOT ONLY DELICIOUS BUT
INSTANTANEOUS.

COFFEE CULTURE

'...coffee is bitter – a flavour from the forbidden and dangerous realm.' Diane Ackermann, *A Natural History of the Senses*

The most popular beverage in the world is coffee. More than six billion pounds of the stuff are traded each year. Once known to Persians and Arabs as the drink of the gods, coffee has now become so much a part of modern life that many people dread to be without it. If you're going to drink coffee, there are certain things you need to know about it. For instance, you should know how to choose the best coffee and how to protect yourself from the contamination from pesticides and herbicides it carries. **(For the Inside Story on coffee, see page 95.)**

The art of making coffee

How do you prepare it? There are many ways. Dyed-in-the-wool coffee lovers who fear the dangers of drinking coffee sometimes make an acid-free coffee extract by putting a pound of freshly ground organic coffee in 1.5 litres (2 1/2 pints) of water and allowing it to soak for 24 hours in a cool, dark place. Then they filter the extract through a coffee filter, put it into a glass jar and store it in the refrigerator. Each time they want a cup of coffee, they add 2-4 tablespoons of the extract to 250 ml (8 fl oz) of hot water. This creates de-acidified coffee that you can keep in the refrigerator for up to two weeks. A couple of cups of this drink taken once or twice a day should be no problem to anyone who is generally healthy. The only problem with this method is that you will not get the same sense of intensity that is so adored by many coffee worshippers.

You can buy organic coffee in its many different forms and make it conventionally as you would ordinary coffee. Each method for coffee brewing – from cafetière or plunger to the Neapolitan macchinetta, the automatic filter method, espresso, the coffee percolator and even Turkish coffee – works equally well, provided it is carried out according to certain principles.

Making the perfect cup of coffee

* Keep all of your coffee-making equipment clean. Make sure that it's washed thoroughly after you use it each time, otherwise the oils in the grounds become rancid and contaminate the fresh brew.

* Always warm a pot before brewing – except, of course, when using methods where you are heating the pot itself in the process.

* Always use the purest of water.

* Always use the right sized grounds for the method you've chosen.

* Drink coffee as soon as it is made – coffee degrades very quickly and takes on negative effects when it's allowed to sit on the hob and keep warm.

* Finally, use *enough* coffee. Generally speaking about 2 tablespoons of ground coffee for each cup works well.

One of the ironies of coffee making is the false notion that people have about espresso. Espresso, which is believed to be so strong, is made from *Coffea arabica*, which happens to be the most widely cultivated coffee in the world and makes up about 75 percent of all the coffees you'll find in shops. Most people believe that espresso, which is thought of as very strong coffee – and indeed it is in its aroma and flavour – is also very high in caffeine. In truth, espresso contains from one-half to one-third less caffeine per cup than does robusta, partly because the arabica beans are lower in caffeine. But this is also because the dark roasting, on which the flavour of espresso and all of the other coffees made from it, like cappuccino and macchiato, burns off much of the caffeine content. The darker the roast, the less caffeine is present in the coffee. The one kind of coffee that I would never drink is instant coffee. First, it is very poor in flavour and second, the processes by which it is made often involve the use of chemical solvents, which you certainly want to be without **(see page 95)**.

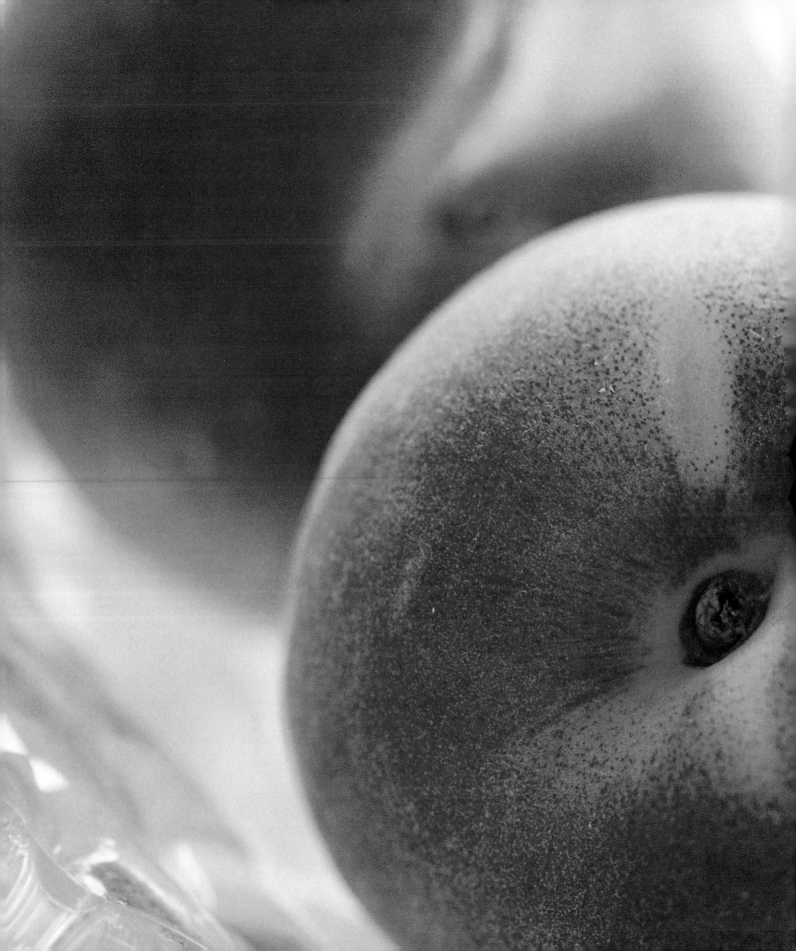

GRAB A PEACH

There is little more wonderful for breakfast than fresh fruit. First, it is easy to digest. Eaten first thing in the morning, fruit helps your body keep right on eliminating the rubbish we all build up, which does us no good, right through the morning. Your liver - the body's organ for cleansing itself - is most active between midnight and midday. If you can manage a breakfast of fruit juice or vegetable juice or a mixture of the two and this is enough for you, more power to you. Your body will just keep on cleansing itself. If not, don't worry. Everybody is unique in his or her needs for breakfast. Whatever you choose for breakfast, provided you don't suffer from Candida albicans, make fruit a part of it. The more colourful the fruit you choose, the better.

The fruit factor

Red, orange and yellow fruits contain a wealth of phytochemical compounds, which not only foster health, but also prevent premature ageing. Some of the most important are called the carotenoids. Studies have shown that they decrease the risk of heart disease, enhance immunity and help prevent macular (retinal) degeneration and many kinds of cancer. So far, more than 600 carotenoids have been identified and many of these - most especially beta-carotene - have been extensively researched for their health-enhancing potential and ability to prevent illness. Each of the carotenoids has a slightly different protective ability.

They tend to work best together, the way they are found in nature. No amount of pill popping will ever replace what you can get from eating fresh fruits as part of your diet.

Alpha-carotene, for example, plays an important role in preventing cellular damage to the liver, the eye and the lungs. Other carotenoids, such as lutein, zeaxanthin and cryptoxanthin, are especially important in preventing cancer and premature ageing. Research shows that eating two or three servings of red, orange or yellow fruits a day - all of which are rich in carotenoids - can reduce your risk of cancer by 50 percent. It can even help protect from damage caused by cigarette smoke. Although most restaurants have non-smoking areas, the dangers to passive smokers, forced to be in a room where others smoke, are far from behind us yet. Another carotenoid, lycopene, is particularly potent in its ability to protect the body from the ravages of time

Every day red, orange and yellow fruits

Raspberries	Watermelons
Strawberries	Cantaloupes
Red grapes	Mangoes
Apricots	Guavas
Peaches	Papayas

Eat it whole

As often as possible eat fruits with the skin on them. The skin of many fruits is an excellent source of pectin. This is the soluble fibre that helps balance blood lipids, stabilize blood sugar and reduce LDL cholesterol (the so-called 'bad' cholesterol as opposed to DHL cholesterol - the 'good' cholesterol). Pectin also encourages the elimination of bile acids in the intestines and reduces toxicity in the body.

Fruits are also rich in vitamin C as well as phenolic acids and flavonoids - all of which have been shown to help prevent premature ageing and heart disease. Raspberries, strawberries and grapes also contain ellagic acid, another ally in keeping your skin firm and unlined and in preventing illness. Apart from the fact that they are incredibly beautiful, a bowl of sliced peaches, a fruit smoothie or a freshly made fruit juice pack a good punch when it comes to looking good and feeling great.

ORANGE CASHEW NECTAR

People avoid raw cashews because they are high in fat. But the fat they contain is good quality - mostly monounsaturates - and easy to digest. Because it digests slowly, it helps keep you from feeling hungry through the morning. These luscious creamy nuts are also rich in magnesium for the nervous system, selenium for free-radical protection and vitamin B1. Mix with a little fresh coconut or coconut milk and fresh orange juice and you turn an instant breakfast into nectar for the gods.

WHAT YOU NEED

250 ml (8 fl oz) orange juice and the flesh of a seeded and peeled orange or 450 ml (16 fl oz) fresh orange juice

25 g (1 oz) raw cashew nuts

2 tbsp fresh coconut, unsweetened coconut cream or dried shredded, unsweetened coconut

maple syrup, honey or rice syrup to taste (optional)

HERE'S HOW

Place the ingredients in a food processor and blend until creamy smooth.

OTHER WAYS TO GO

Nuts to go: Replace the cashews with almonds or hazelnuts, pecans or black walnuts.

Raisins: Replace the coconut with a handful of raisins.

Dates: Replace the honey or rice syrup with a few fresh dates.

JUICE AND THE X-FACTOR

Freshly extracted fruit and vegetable juice are not only delicious, they empower health and good looks like nothing else. Start by taking one glass of whatever mixture you fancy - carrot and apple are a good way to begin - and you will notice amazing things start to happen. First you will find you get a great lift from these radiant liquids. Then you will begin to notice improvement in your skin and in your overall energy levels. You may find that you no longer need a stiff cup of coffee to get you going. Once your body becomes accustomed to drinking raw juices, you may even discover they do it better than coffee and without the energy slumps that many coffee drinkers experience from plunging blood sugar levels at 11am.

Rejuvenating juices

Brightly coloured fruits and vegetables are rampant with plant factors to enhance health and good looks. And they carry a big wallop for vitality simply because the phytonutrients in the plants from which they are made come in a highly concentrated form as juice. But there is something else too about juice - something that nutrition, despite its tremendous advances, still cannot measure. I call it the X-factor. I suppose the closest you can get to describe it is as a natural raw energy that cannot be measured in chemical terms alone. Speak of it and you move out of the realms of biochemistry, breaching the secrets of high level physics. You have to begin talking about light energy - the energy from the sun, from the big bang that 15 billion light years away created the universe, the galaxies, the sun itself. It is the same energy from which our bodies are made and the same energy that plants absorb and, through photosynthesis, partly convert to chemical compounds we can identify for health and good looks.

The ability of raw juices to regenerate and rejuvenate the body in medically measurable ways has been long known and is in no small part because it carries this potent life force. The famous Rohsaft Kur - raw juice, sure - developed

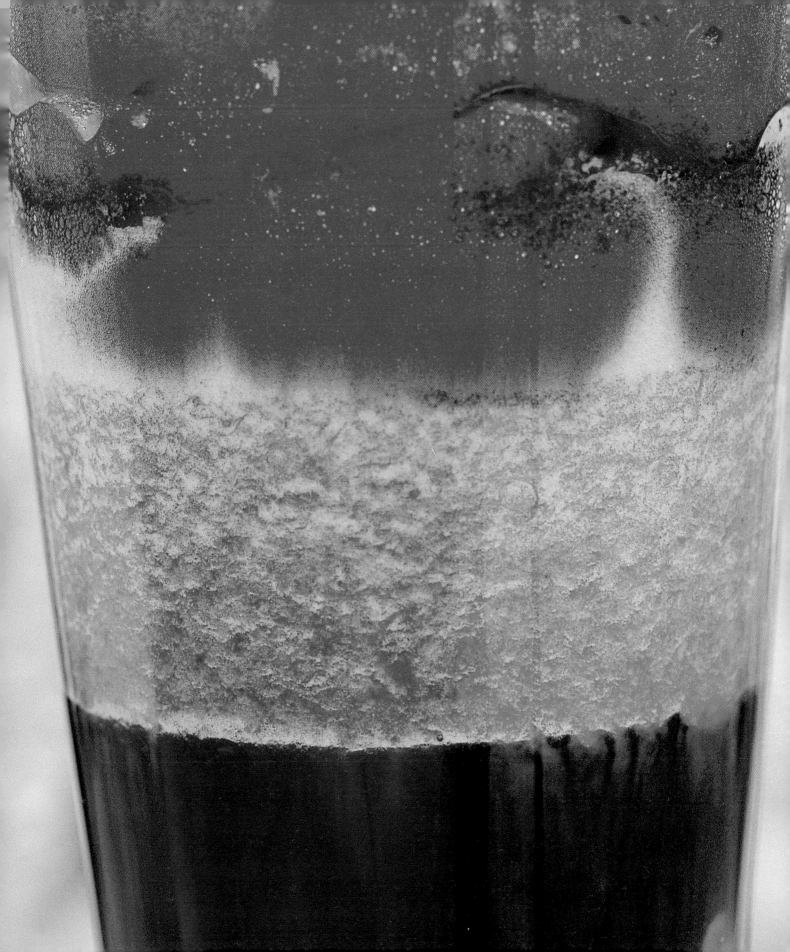

by European doctors like Max Bircher-Benner and Max Gerson almost a century ago is now acknowledged by natural medicine to be the single most potent short-term antidote to fatigue and stress. Until recently, it has been the preserve of the privileged few who can afford to go to exclusive spas and health farms. Now, thanks to the coming of affordable centrifugal juicers, which are a lot easier to clean than their expensive predecessors, fresh fruits and vegetable juices are available in our homes.

Drunk daily for breakfast or whenever you need a refreshing break during the day, their goodness is delivered direct to your system, bringing a synergistic range of nutrients and X-factor energy, including the living energy of enzymes to replenish whatever is lacking in your body. If you are not familiar with juice-drinking, begin with fruit juices. Then move on to vegetable juices by starting with half apple and half carrot and gradually add the green juices from celery, spinach and maybe dandelion or some powerful beetroot juice. But go easy. Juices are more powerful than you first imagine and it takes time for most people to develop a taste for the wilder flavours that various plants impart. Here are a few of my favourite fruit juice combinations. All can be made in a juice extractor by following the manufacturer's instructions. Try a few and see what you like best. Then you can make up your own.

Favourite fruit juices

Raspberry topped with apple
Apple and pear
Orange and pink grapefruit
Cranberry and grape
Peach and tangerine
Papaya and strawberries
Grape, berries and 12 mm
   (1/2 in) piece of fresh
   ginger
Watermelon

Fruit and vegetable juices

Carrot and apple
Carrot, apple, beetroot and
   broccoli
Tomato, celery and pineapple
   plus 1 tsp to 1 tbsp of
   Spirulina powder
Apple and celery
Pineapple with a few leaves of
   fresh mint
1/2 melon, flesh of 1 lime and
   12 mm (1/2 in) piece of
   fresh ginger

GET INTO SOYA

I'm a great proponent of soya. First, there is so much that you can do with it. Second, in the wake of all the research that has taken place in the last ten years into the powerful, protective properties of the soya bean, this humble food has a significant contribution to make to our health, energy and good looks. That is, provided the source of soya you are using comes from beans that have not been genetically engineered.

Dare to avoid dairy products

With the exception of the odd bit of shredded Parmesan and the use of butter, you will find no dairy products within these pages. There is a good reason for this. Many people – usually unbeknown to them - are food sensitive to the protein in milk, cheese, yoghurt and cream. Butter escapes this list because it is not a dairy protein but a fat. In fact, butter is a very useful food – provided you do not use far too much of it. Milk proteins tend to create mucus in the body and, in people who are milk sensitive or 'allergic', eating them can make you highly prone to fatigue and weight gain, aches and pains and even the development of many degenerative conditions. So widespread is the sensitivity to milk that an amazing 70 percent of the population of the world is affected by it.

The best source of calcium is actually green vegetables and cereal grasses – where the cows themselves get their own calcium. It is more readily assimilated than the calcium in cows' milk and comes packaged with magnesium and other elements essential to building and preserving strong bones. One of the great ironies about how we need to take more dairy products and take calcium supplements to prevent osteoporosis, is that statistics show that in the United States – where the consumption of milk and calcium as an element is highest in the world – so is the incidence of osteoporosis. In China, where almost no milk products are used and the calcium intake from green vegetables is only moderate, the incidence of osteoporosis is lowest. Soya is a good alternative. (For the Inside Story on soya, see page 94.)

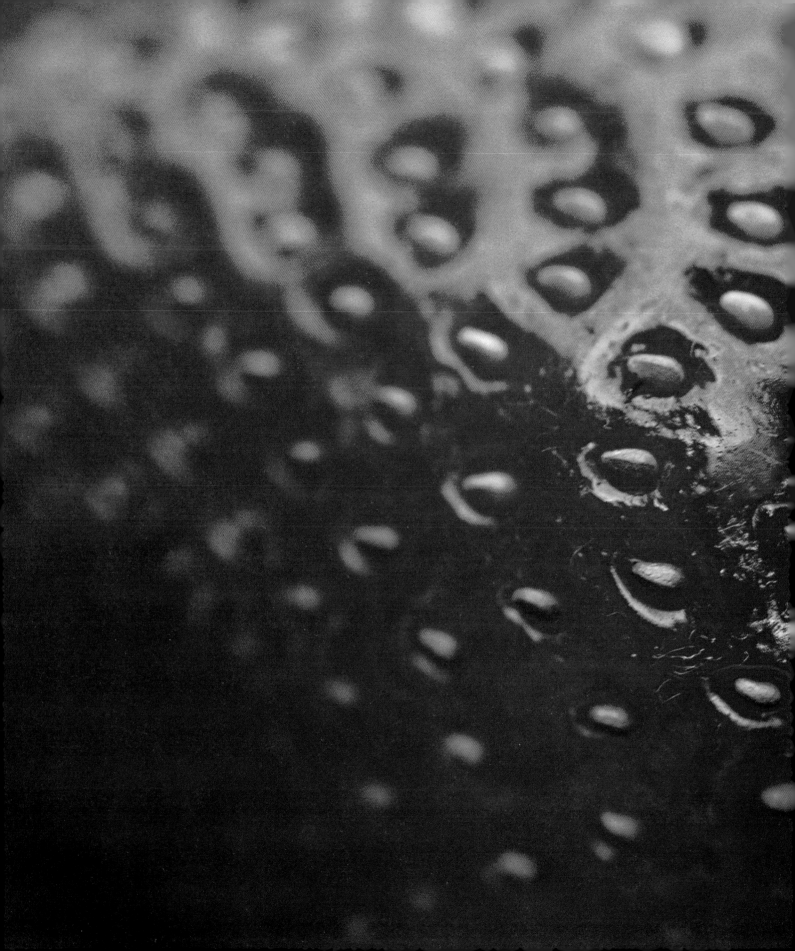

STRAWBERRY PROTECTOR

This is an instant breakfast, full of minerals and vitamins. High in fibre and low in fat, it is also rich in potassium and in the plant hormones that help protect men from a lowered sperm count and women from reproductive disorders such as PMS, fibroids and osteoporosis. All you need to make it is a food processor. It has many variations, all of them delicious. I use whatever fruits I happen to have available. (For the Inside Story on bananas, see page 84.)

WHAT YOU NEED
375 ml (12 fl oz) soya milk
100 g (4 oz) fresh or frozen
   strawberries
1 ripe medium banana, peeled
   and sliced
2 tbsp oat bran
1 tsp vanilla extract
pinch of nutmeg

HERE'S HOW
Put everything into a food processor except the nutmeg and mix until thick and smooth. Before serving, sprinkle with a little nutmeg.

OTHER WAYS TO GO

Applejack: Replace the strawberries with 2 fresh apples and add cinnamon to the top.

Pineapple delight: Replace the strawberries with fresh pineapple and blend together with 3 or 4 leaves of fresh mint.

Blueberry shake: Use a large handful of blueberries in place of the strawberries. Top with chopped almonds.

Spiced mango lassi: Process a handful of cashews with 250 ml (8 fl oz) soya milk, 2 mangoes and some cinnamon, cardamom, nutmeg and honey to taste. (For the Inside Story on mangoes, see page 86.)

MOCK JULIUS

serves 1

When I was a kid, there was nothing I liked better than the American drink Orange Julius. But, like lots of things children love, it had a few things in it that it's better not to eat – like sugar syrup. This is my own recipe. It is quite different from the original, yet inspired by its deliciousness.

WHAT YOU NEED

3 oranges, peeled, sliced and seeded
1 raw organic or free-range egg
2 tbsp maple syrup or 1 tbsp liquid honey
3 tbsp organic soya milk powder or vanilla-flavoured micro-filtered whey protein powder
1 tsp vanilla extract
6 ice cubes

HERE'S HOW

Combine all the ingredients in a food processor. Whirl at high speed for a minute or two, just until frothy. Drink immediately.

FIBRE MATTERS

Fresh fruits and vegetables are full of fibre, both soluble and insoluble. So are grains and pulses. However, the fibre in fresh vegetables – particularly when they are eaten raw – acts quite differently from the fibre in cooked beans, breads, cereals and pasta. It is easier on the body and works better to help detoxify it in an on-going way. Thank heaven the idea that wheat bran is something everybody should get lots and lots of for health is beginning to fade. The truth, for many, is that taking extra wheat bran causes constipation. It can be highly irritating to the bowel.

Fibre fine points

If you want to add extra cereal fibres, one of the best ways to go is to eat oat bran. It tastes good, makes a great hot cereal or adjunct to porridge, is useful in baking scones and bread, and is soothing to the gut. If you are someone who has been living for a long time on a diet of convenience foods, be sure to add more cooked fibre from grains or pulses slowly into your life; otherwise it can shock your system and you may end up with digestive disturbances until your body adjusts. When it comes to introducing fibres from fresh fruits and vegetables, this is not the case. Most people can change over from a low-fibre diet to a high-fibre one this way much more quickly without distress. For a list of the different fibres and how they work wonders for health **see the Inside Story on page 89.**

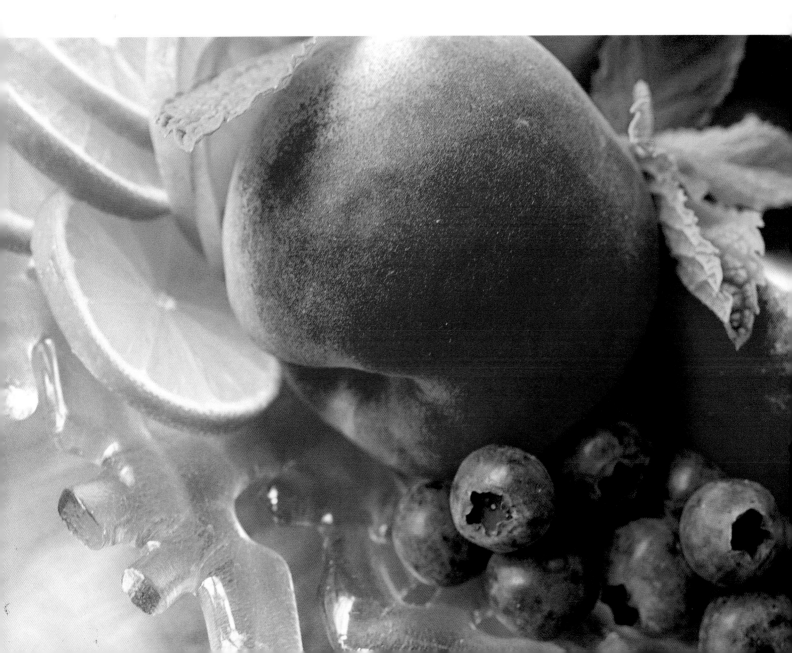

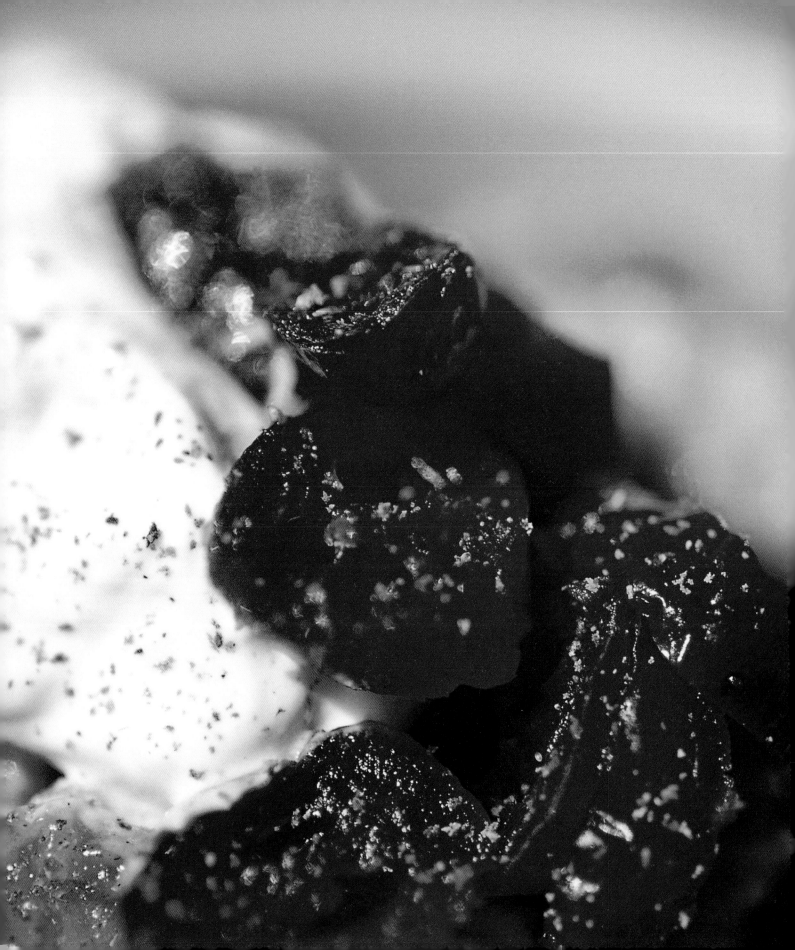

INSTANT CRANBERRY PORRIDGE

When I know I will want an instant breakfast, I like to make porridge the night before. Oat porridge is a great way to start the day. It carries the kind of slow carbohydrate energy that is steadily released into your body throughout the morning. This breakfast is particularly good if you are someone who just does not function on juice or fruit alone. (For the Inside Story on cranberries, see page 86.)

WHAT YOU NEED

25 g (1 oz) dried cranberries
25 g (1 oz) rolled oats
1 tsp honey or concentrated apple or pear juice
375 ml (12 fl oz) boiling water
1/4 tsp cinnamon or freshly ground nutmeg
1 tsp butter (optional)

HERE'S HOW

Put all the ingredients except the cinnamon or nutmeg and butter into a Thermos and close. Set aside until morning. You can also use a Pyrex jar with a lid that closes and place it in a warm place, such as the warming oven of an Aga, through the night. Eat as is, sprinkled with cinnamon or nutmeg and topped with butter (if you want), or cover with soya milk, oat milk or rice milk. You can vary the porridge you make by using other grain flakes such as barley, millet or brown rice flakes.

OTHER WAYS TO GO

Date dream: Use a large handful of chopped and pitted dates instead of the cranberries.

Fruit on hand: Make the porridge without fruit then, just before eating it, add a handful of fresh or frozen berries, a sliced banana, a grated apple or whatever else you can find.

GET BRUNCHED

2

The smell of oranges and the
crunch of fresh linen as light
slips through the window. It
happens seldom - only on special
Sundays. Time for brunch. A
luscious, languid meal with
friends, brunch needs to be
spiked with surprises: Bloody
Mary made with fresh tomato
juice served with omelette
topped with Mexican salsa or
perhaps the sweet innocence of
Bircher Muesli made with
strawberries or fresh mangoes.
Consume fresh lavender muffins
replete with flowers from the
garden in summer and in winter
plan for stir-fried leeks and
wild mushrooms.

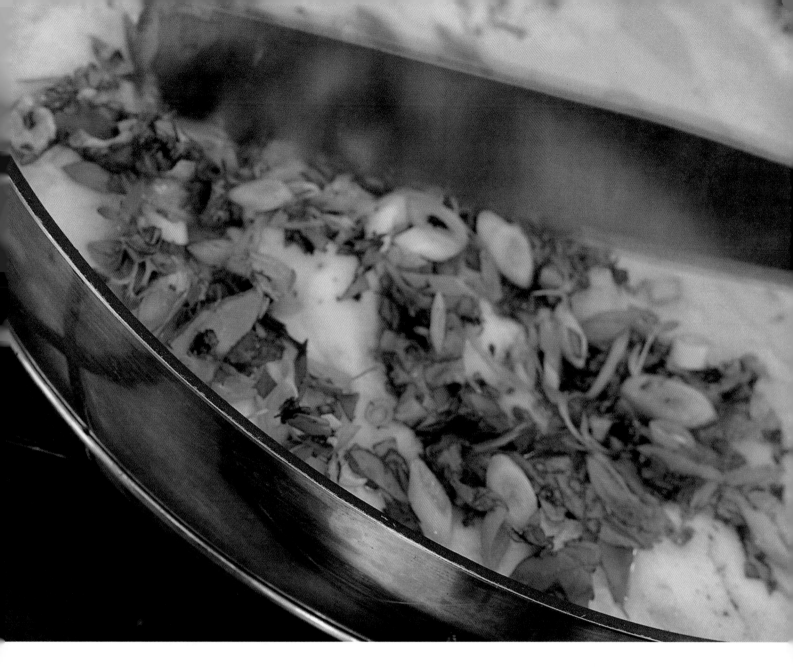

A TIME FOR GATHERING, FOR CELEBRATING, FOR INDULGENCE,
BRUNCH IS COMMUNAL, RELAXED, INVENTIVE —

SHEER BLISS

THE PERFECT BRUNCH

makes 2 glasses

VIRGIN MARY/BLOODY MARY

This drink bears little resemblance to the familiar Bloody Mary made with canned tomato juice. You can serve it virgin style – straight up – or add a little vodka to give it a kick. I like to pour it over crushed ice in the summer and serve it in a flared, rimmed, long-stemmed goblet. In winter, I serve it at room temperature in a tall glass.

For generations tomatoes were thought of as a poisonous fruit. In fact, they were once called mala insana – 'unhealthy fruit'. As far back as the seventeenth century, they were thought to provoke not only upset stomachs but also a sense of loathing in anyone who ate them. As it turns out, only the French, who refer to tomatoes as pommes d'amour or 'love apples', got it right. Far from being poisonous, tomatoes are rich in health-enhancing compounds, including high levels of vitamin C, lycopene and many other, probably as yet unidentified, compounds. (For the Inside Story on tomatoes, see page 88.)

WHAT YOU NEED
3 ripe tomatoes
1 stalk of celery (leaves and
   all if they are fresh)
1 medium carrot
60 ml (2 fl oz) vodka
   (optional)
a dash of Tabasco or
   Worcestershire sauce
Maldon sea salt and freshly
   ground pepper
Cajun seasoning (see page 43) or
   grated horseradish
6 ice cubes

HERE'S HOW
Place the tomatoes, celery and carrot in a juice extractor. Then mix with the vodka, if you are using it, season and serve immediately over ice to preserve the living enzymes in the juice and the flavour. You can also make this drink in a food processor without the ice, but this makes it more a spooning drink than a drinking one.

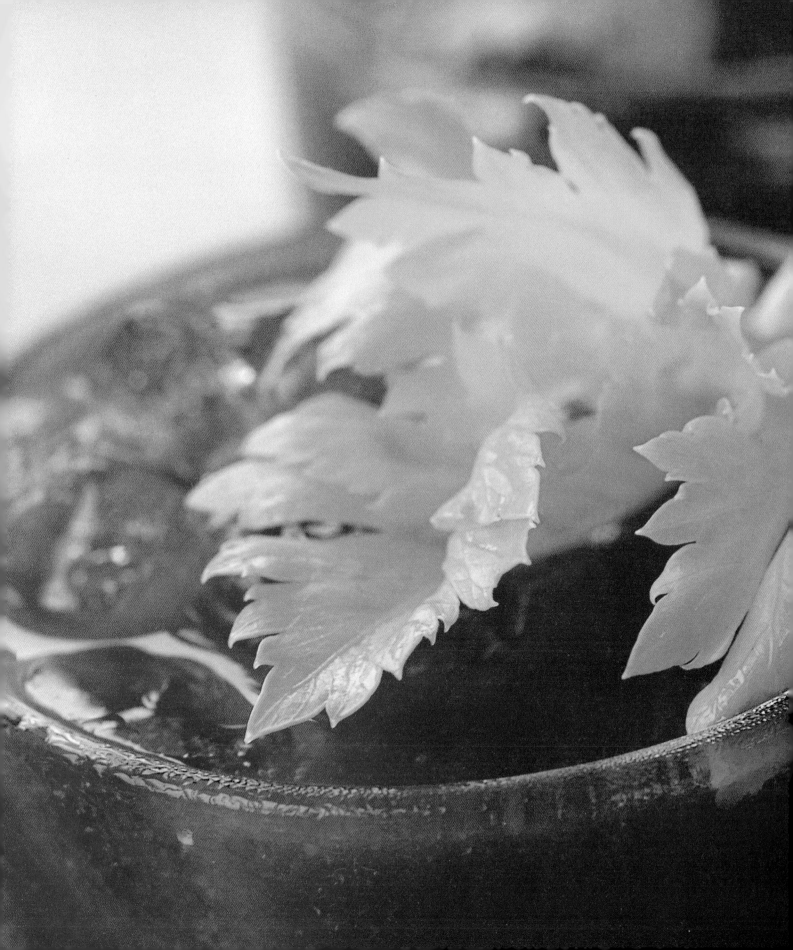

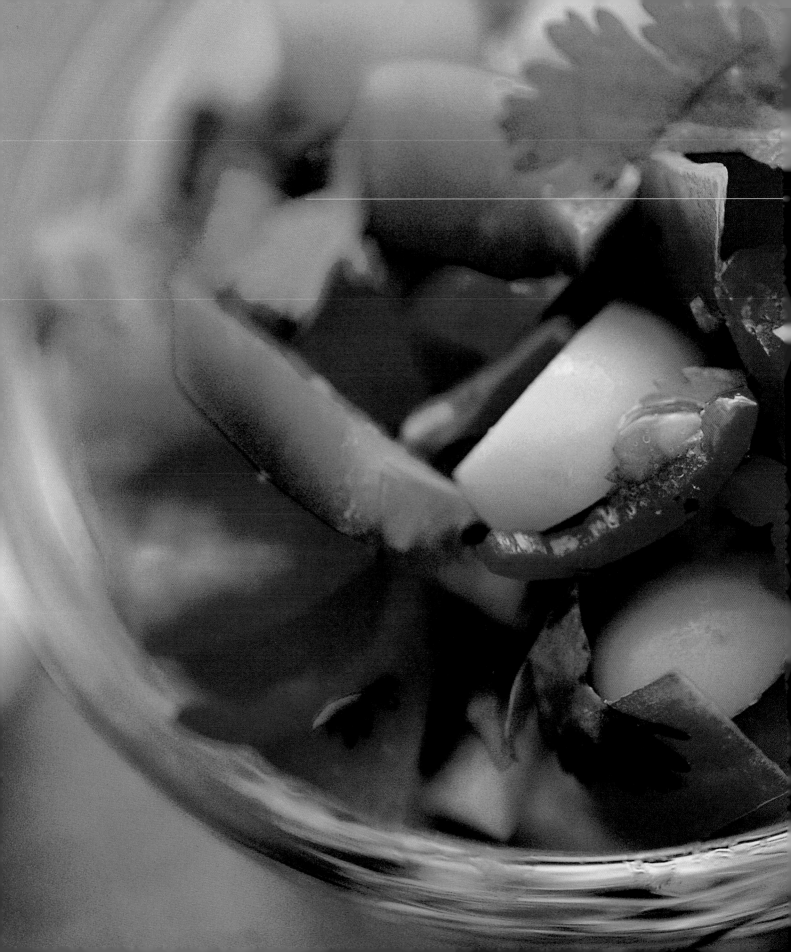

ENERGY SALSA

Delicious salsas and relishes have replaced many of the heavy sauces of the past. They are low in fat — sometimes even fat free — piquant and a great way to add zing to anything from cooked vegetables and tortilla chips to fish and jacket potatoes. You can even eat them on rice or pasta. It used to be that salsas were served cold. Now you'll find them atop cooked dishes as well. I like to serve this salsa on omelettes for brunch, or at other meals with crudités or as a topping for a baked potato.

This recipe is a true energy food. Raw, it needs to be made fresh and will keep for no more than 24 hours in the refrigerator. Go easy on the chillies. You can always add more. But if you go overboard there is nothing you can do to reinstate the coolness of the vegetables afterwards. I like to cut my salsas rougher than most so you get a wonderful mixture of textures as well as flavours. Make them in a food processor and to my mind they end up more like a soup than a salsa. (For the Inside Story on chillies, see page 90.)

WHAT YOU NEED
2 garlic cloves, finely chopped
1 large red onion, chopped
handful of fresh coriander,
    chopped
handful of fresh basil or 2
    tbsp fresh mint, chopped
handful of broad-leaf parsley,
    chopped
green or red chilli pepper,
    roughly chopped
250 g (9 oz) firm tomatoes,
    roughly chopped
1 large green pepper, roughly
    chopped
Maldon sea salt and freshly
    ground pepper
3 tbsp extra-virgin olive oil
3 tbsp lemon or lime juice

HERE'S HOW
Combine all the ingredients in a serving bowl, season and let the mixture sit in the refrigerator for 15 minutes so the flavours meld. Serve immediately or keep it in the refrigerator for up to a day.

LAVENDER MUFFINS

Lavender is the queen of great European herbs. The very best for eating is English lavender *Lavandula angustifolia* or *Lavendula vera*. It is hardier than the French lavender with its blunt, narrow, grey-green leaves. It also has the finest fragrance and flavour. However you use it - to fragrance your laundry or improve the flavour and beauty of muffins - the fragrant flowers of this shrubby plant calms the mind and strengthens the spirit.

Put lavender together with oat bran and you have a wonderful combination. Oat bran is the outer layer of the oat groat - the hulled whole kernel. It helps lower blood cholesterol, probably because it boasts a higher percentage of water-soluble fibre than any other cereal grain bran. Oat bran also appears to be useful in clearing various substances from the body which contribute to high blood cholesterol levels. These muffins are rich in fibre yet contain no wheat. They go well with teas, herb teas and instant liquid breakfasts. The golden granulated sugar included in this recipe is the only truly unrefined sugar. It is processed at a low temperature to preserve its organic acids, enzymes and other nutritional values (see Resources).

WHAT YOU NEED

1 apple, cored and chopped
2 tbsp melted butter
1 egg
1 tsp grated orange rind
1 tsp ground cinnamon
   (optional)
2 tbsp golden granulated sugar
   (optional)
175 ml (6 fl oz) soya milk
100 g (4 oz) oat bran
1 tbsp dried lavender flowers
2 tsp baking powder

HERE'S HOW

Preheat the oven to 200°C/ 400°F/Gas Mark 6. Lightly oil a standard muffin tin. Put the first seven ingredients into a food processor and mix until well combined. Put the oat bran, lavender flowers and baking powder into a separate bowl and pour in the liquid mixture. Stir together until the mixtures are just blended. Two-thirds fill each muffin tin and bake for 15 to 20 minutes in the middle of the oven. Remove and allow to cool in the tin before turning out.

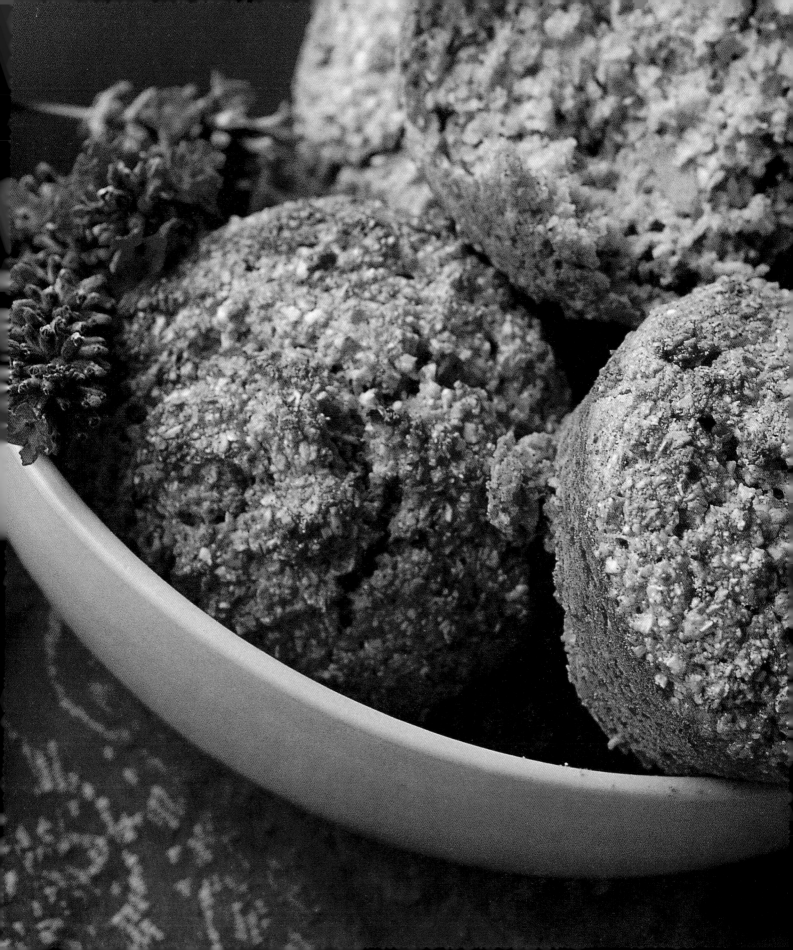

BIRCHER MUESLI

When it comes to health and good looks, nothing carries the power of fresh raw foods. Not only are they higher in essential nutrients than their cooked counterparts, the quality of the nutraceuticals or phytochemicals they contain is the best in the world. Contrary to what a lot of people think, raw fruits and vegetables are also easy to digest. Each fruit or vegetable, fish or seed carries within it the exact enzymes necessary for us to digest it efficiently and fully.

Bircher Muesli was created by the great Swiss physician Max Bircher-Benner, who first healed himself of what was apparently an incurable condition using a high-raw diet and then went on to heal hundreds of thousands of others in the same way. Bircher Muesli is so delicious that even dyed-in-the-wool junk-food eaters fall for it. If you are using dried fruits, be sure to soak them overnight in spring water so that they plump up. Choose whatever fruit is inexpensive and in season.

WHAT YOU NEED
2 tbsp oat flakes (or a combination of oat, rye and wheat), soaked overnight in a little spring water or fruit juice
handful of raisins, also soaked overnight
1 apple or fresh apricot, grated or chopped
juice of 1/2 lemon
3 tbsp soya milk or low-fat plain yoghurt
1 tbsp concentrated apple, pear or strawberry juice
1/4 tsp powdered cinnamon or grated fresh ginger

HERE'S HOW
Mix together the soaked oat flakes and raisins and combine this mixture with the grated or chopped apple or apricot, lemon juice and the soya milk or low-fat yoghurt. Drizzle with concentrated fruit juice and sprinkle with cinnamon or ginger. Serve immediately.

OTHER WAYS TO GO

Winter muesli: Soak a selection of dried fruit such as apricots, sultanas, figs, dates and pears, overnight in spring water. Dice into small pieces or cut up with scissors and add to the soaked grain flakes. Add the lemon juice, soya milk or yoghurt and concentrated fruit juice. Spice with a little grated nutmeg.

Fruit juice muesli: Substitute some fresh fruit juice, such as apple, orange or grape, for the soya milk or yoghurt. To thicken the juice, blend with a little fresh fruit in season such as banana, pear or apple.

Banana muesli: Add a banana sliced in quarters lengthways and then chopped crosswise into small pieces, or mash a banana with a little soya milk, yoghurt or fruit juice and use it as a topping. Summer muesli: Add a handful of raisins, strawberries, blackcurrants or pitted cherries to the basic muesli, or substitute a finely diced peach or nectarine for the apple.

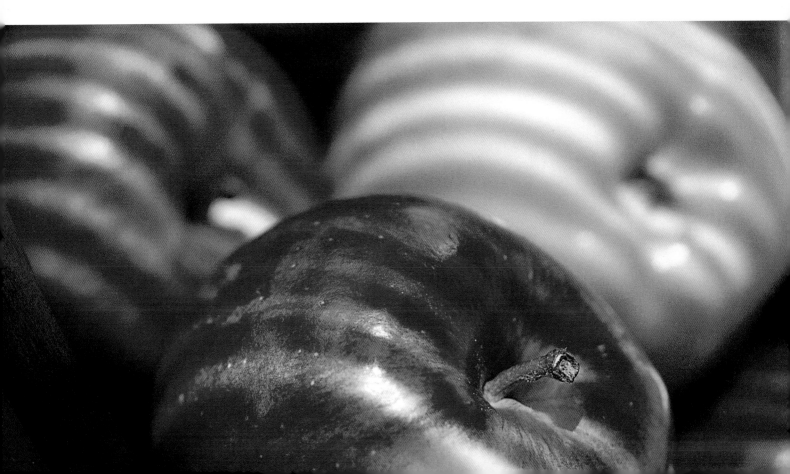

MUSHROOMS ARE MAGIC

If you still think of mushrooms as nothing more than a garnish for a dish or a 'must' for pizza in between the grilled cheese, it's time to think again. Recent studies show that - just as the Chinese have been claiming for the last 7,000 years - most of the more than 35,000 different varieties of fungi have health-enhancing abilities. Even the common button mushrooms, which do not yet appear to have specific healing properties, are an excellent source of B complex vitamins, especially pantothenic acid, which helps enhance your body's ability to deal with stress, as well as niacin, riboflavin and the elusive vitamin B12. In fact, so rich are button mushrooms in vitamin B12, that just three of these tiny gifts from nature are enough to help you meet the recommended daily allowance for this nutrient, which is essential for brain and nerve health. Mushrooms are also rich in potassium and in iron. (For the Inside Story on mushrooms, see page 87.)

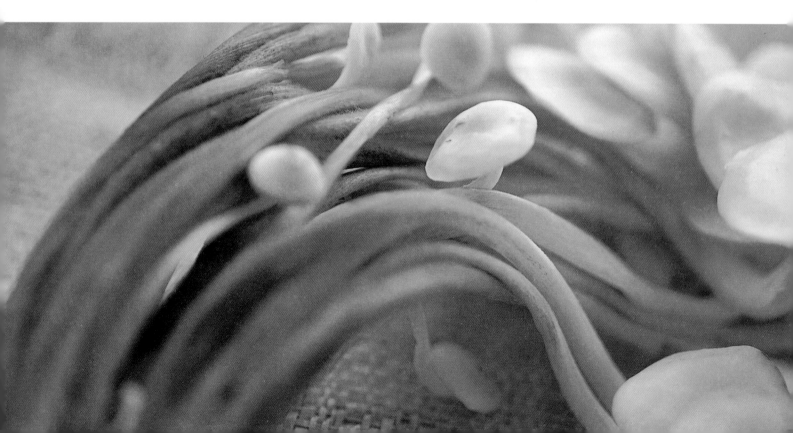

serves 4

WILD MUSHROOM SALAD

Easy to make, delicious and health-enhancing, wild mushroom salad is a winner at brunch, lunch or tea. I like to mix wild mushrooms with shiitaki, reishi and maitake mushrooms, which I buy fresh if I can. As often as not I am forced to use the dry ones instead. Dried mushrooms are easy to prepare. Pop them into a pot and cover them with water then bring them to the boil and simmer for 15 to 20 minutes. Drain the mushrooms. Now they are ready for use in any recipe.

WHAT YOU NEED

250 g (9 oz) mixed salad
   leaves, according to
   whatever is in season
300 g (10 oz) wild mushrooms,
   washed and dried, or dried
   mushrooms, prepared as above
25 g (1 oz) butter
2 tbsp extra-virgin olive oil
125 ml (4 fl oz) dry white
   wine
pinch of saffron threads
lean vinaigrette dressing **(see
   page 184)**
Maldon sea salt and freshly
   ground pepper
fresh coriander or other fresh
   herbs, e.g. basil or broad-
   leaved parsley, to garnish

HERE'S HOW

Clean the salad leaves and dry either in a tea towel or in a basket. Pop them into the refrigerator to crisp up. Slice the mushrooms and, if you're going to cook them, fry very quickly in the butter and olive oil over a gentle heat, just until they begin to look juicy. Then add the wine and the saffron to help the flavours combine. Remove from the heat and cool. If you're going to use the mushrooms raw, wash and slice them and, after reconstituting any dried mushrooms you are going to use, you're ready to go. Put the salad leaves into the bowl and toss with a light vinaigrette dressing, then add the mushrooms and pour on the rest of the dressing. Add some Maldon sea salt and very coarsely ground black pepper to season, add the other herbs to garnish and serve.

GRIND YOUR OWN

I have never met a pepper grinder I didn't hate. Even the ones that work when you buy them seem to give out before long. That is what got me into grinding my pepper corns the old-fashioned way with mortar and pestle. That too is how I discovered what a profound difference there is in pepper ground by hand this way. The essential oils of the spice flood into the air from the surface of the freshly broken-up pepper, in turn flooding your senses while you are performing the act.

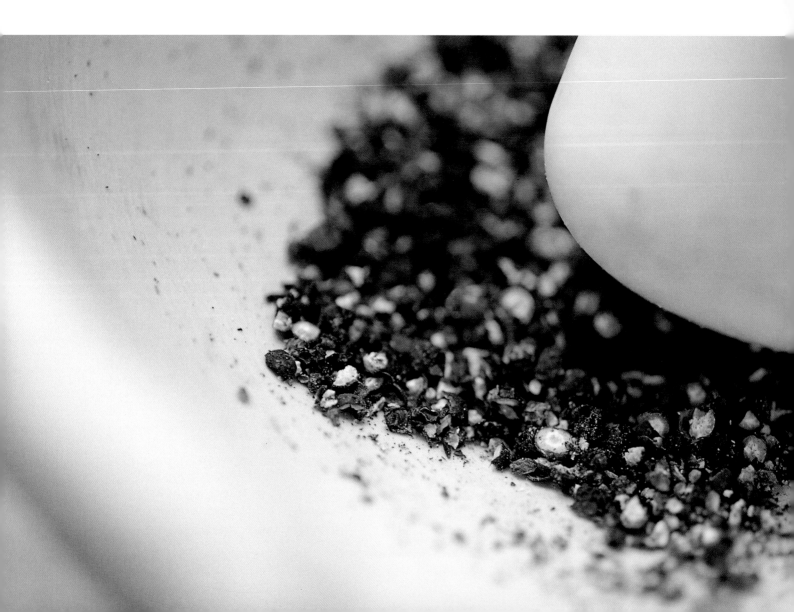

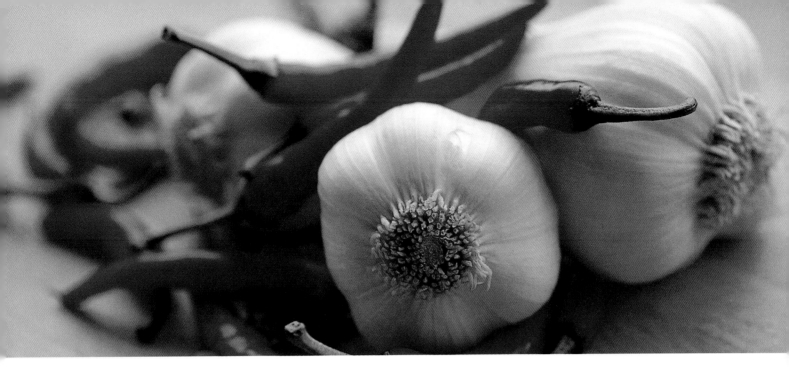

HOMEMADE CAJUN SEASONING

This recipe comes from my friend Shirley Bradstock, who did the cooking for all the photos I shot for this book. She is a passionate and energetic woman who was shocked to see that I use powdered Cajun seasoning from the supermarket. She insisted that I become converted to making my own. It is best made with fresh herbs and fresh onions and garlic and you can then keep it in the refrigerator for up to two weeks. If you want a dry mixture that will keep longer, use dried garlic and onion flakes instead.

WHAT YOU NEED
1 tsp paprika
1/2 tsp freshly ground pepper
1/2 tsp ground cumin
1/2 tsp mustard powder
1/2 tsp cayenne pepper
2 tsp fresh thyme or 1/2 tsp
   dried thyme
1 tsp Maldon sea salt
2 tsp fresh oregano or 1 tsp
   dried oregano
2-3 garlic cloves, well mashed
1 chilli, finely chopped
3 tbsp grated onion

HERE'S HOW
Combine all ingredients by hand. Store in a jar with a tightly closing lid. Use immediately or keep in the refrigerator for up to two weeks if you have used fresh herbs, or several weeks if you have used dried.

CRUNCHY FEASTS

3

The quickest and easiest way to change your life for the better is to add more salads. Forget the limp lettuce leaf and tomato fare. We're talking rich green mesclun and brilliant flowers, wild herbs, fennel and orange with mangetout tendrils, bright peppers, brilliant Swiss chard and almonds – crunchy, delicious and a snap to make. Salads brimming with phytonutrients to detoxify your body, protect from premature ageing and energize your life. Salad making is far more an art than a science. I am always amused by people who say they love salads but just don't have time to make them. I can create a salad that is a whole meal for four people and have it

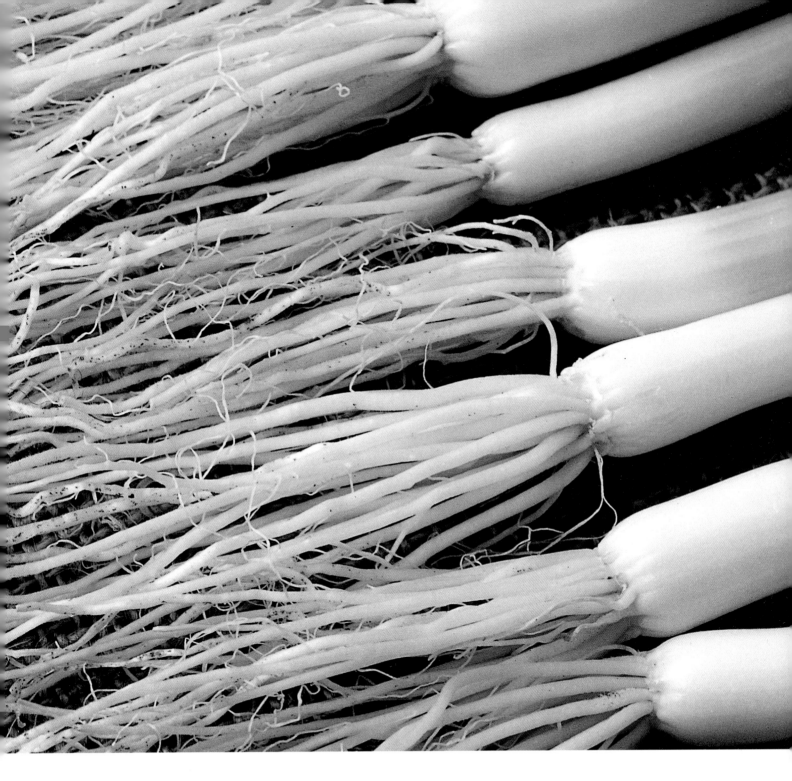

ON THE TABLE IN 10 MINUTES.

FOR THE LOVE OF SALADS

Salad making begins at the shopping stage: buy what is most beautiful and forget the rest. Bring home your vegetables, wash them thoroughly and dry them. Then place them ready-to-use in vegetable bins in the refrigerator. Shop for fresh vegetables a couple of times a week and do this as soon as you get home, then you are all set for instant salads. The hardest part about making a salad is simply getting your vegetables ready to use and when all of this is done at one time in advance. The putting together of these beautiful bright-coloured gifts from nature becomes a kind of blissful meditation. I love working with whatever is there. You can make a fabulous salad from a beetroot and a couple of apples grated using a mandolin then topped with fresh orange juice, a handful of chopped herbs and some curry powder. It is that easy.

Get a textural balance

The one piece of equipment I would never be without is a mandolin. Here you see the gorgeous (and expensive) stainless steel variety. It is good and oh so beautiful but to tell you the truth I prefer the simple plastic ones that sell for a fifth of the price. They have a v-shaped blade into which plastic inserts fit, each of which has different-sized knives so you can julienne, make chip-sized chunks, slice thin or thick. Unlike the conventional grater, which mashes vegetables and fruits when you use it, a mandolin slices them clean and sharp. Be sure to use the hand-protecting device that comes with either model. If you don't - and I know from experience - what you will end up with is shredded fingers instead of shredded cabbage.

I try to mix between two and five vegetables (sometimes fruits too) to make a salad. Not only do I mix vegetables, I also mix textures - using a finely julienned carrot together with a coarsely grated apple and celery perhaps plus some slivered spring onions. It is the mixture of colour and textures that make it all work.

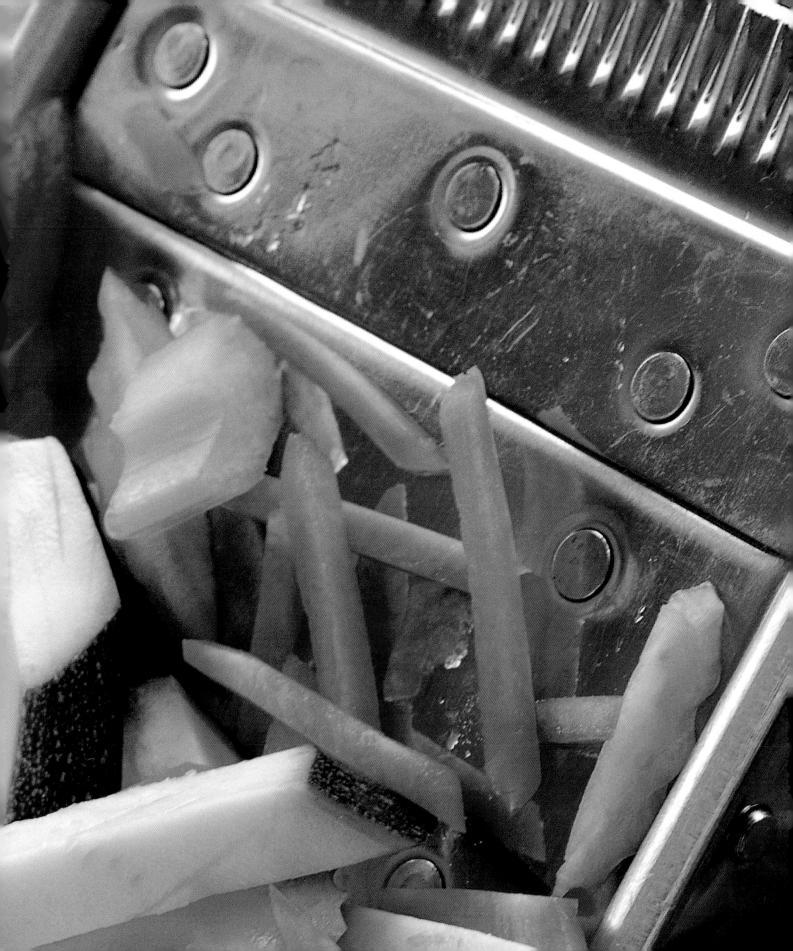

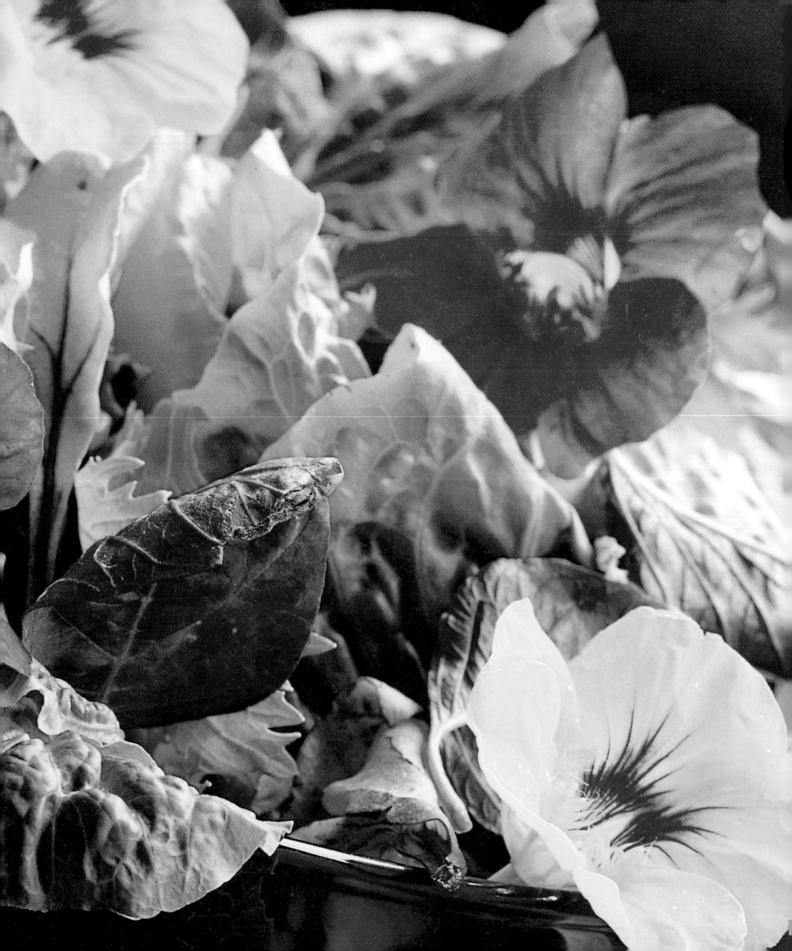

MESCLUN AND FLOWER SALAD

serves 4

A French Provençal word, 'mesclun' means a mixture of delicate salad leaves, including such things as curly endive, romaine, red radicchio, flat-leaved parsley, dandelions - even purslane. These leaves are not only easy to grow, most are harvested by cutting a few at a time and allowing the plants to get on reproducing yet more beautiful leaves. You can buy mesclun to grow in your own garden. It comes in packages of seeds called 'saladisi'; or buy one of the 'cut-and-come-again' salad varieties.

WHAT YOU NEED
3 or 4 of any of the following
  mesclun leaves:
  curly endive
  dandelion leaves
  lamb's lettuce
  oak-leaf lettuce
  purslane
  red radicchio
  rocket
  romaine lettuce
  10-12 brightly coloured
  nasturtium flowers

FOR THE DRESSING
2 garlic cloves, finely chopped
1/4 tsp Dijon mustard
4 tbsp walnut oil
1 tbsp white wine vinegar
1 tbsp chervil, finely chopped
1 tbsp flat-leaved parsley,
  finely chopped

HERE'S HOW
Put all the mesclun leaves into a huge glass salad bowl - I use glass because the leaves are so beautiful that it's a shame to conceal them. Then, for the dressing, put all the ingredients into a screw-topped jar and shake vigorously to blend. Sprinkle over the leaves and toss very lightly and serve immediately. This is a very delicate salad, and like all delicate things, it needs careful handling to prevent bruising.

serves 4

FENNEL, ORANGE AND GRAPE SALAD

The fresh, crunchy taste of fennel makes you feel as though it's good for you when you eat it, and indeed it is. Sodium and potassium are antagonists – they need to be taken in by the body in good balance **in order to maintain health. Most of us eat too much salt – sodium chloride. Fennel, which is rich in potassium, helps redress the imbalance.** (For the Inside Story on fennel, see page 87.)

WHAT YOU NEED
2 medium-sized bulbs of fennel
2 large or 4 small ripe
   oranges
125 ml (8 fl oz) mangetout
   tendrils
175 g (6 oz) black and/or
   white grapes, removed from
   the stalk

DRESSING
2 tbsp walnut oil
1 tsp Meaux mustard
1 tbsp chopped broad-leaved
   parsley
1 garlic clove, finely chopped
Maldon sea salt and freshly
   ground pepper

HERE'S HOW
Slice the fennel crosswise so that you end up with oval-shaped pieces. Peel the orange and break into slices. Add all of these to a flat bowl and garnish with the mangetout tendrils and grapes. For the dressing, put everything into a jar. Shake it up and pour it over the salad. Toss and serve immediately on separate plates.

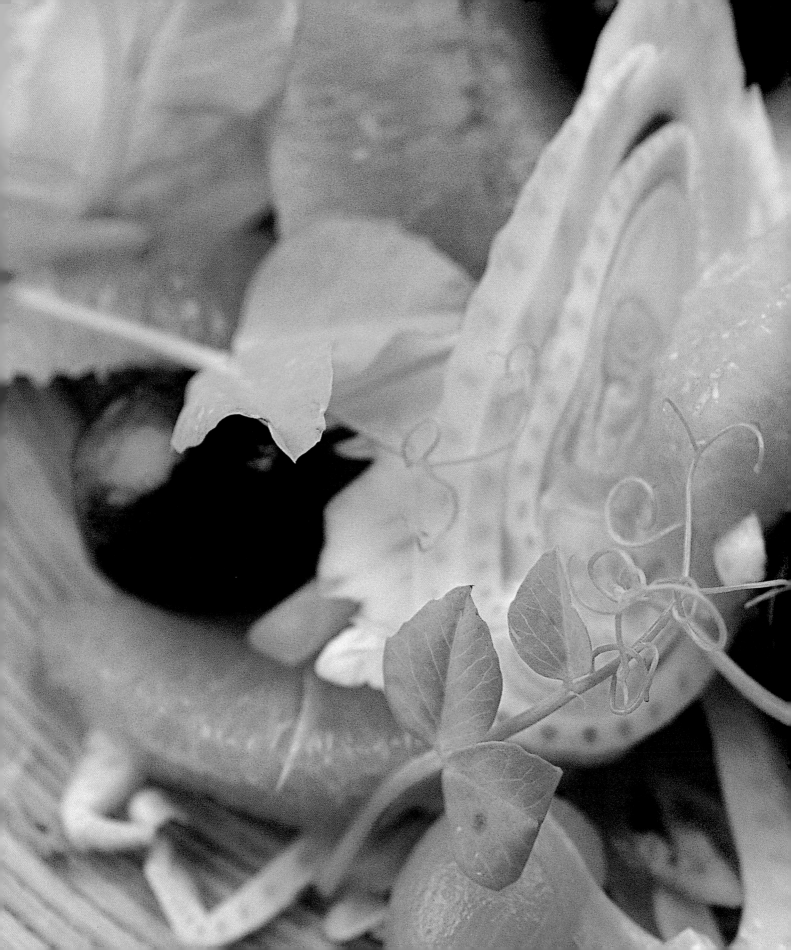

CAESAR SALAD WITH POTATO CROUTONS

Add something surprising to a salad or do it your own way. One day, I hit upon the idea of making potato croutons for a wheat-free Caesar salad. Crispy oven-baked gems with traditional Caesar dressing complete with a raw, free-range, organic egg is great. But don't try to make this dressing with a battery egg; for there is always the possibility of salmonella. (For the Inside Story on anchovies and eggs, see pages 92 and 94.)

WHAT YOU NEED FOR THE SALAD

2 heads of romaine lettuce
100 g (4 oz) Parmesan cheese, shaved not grated
12 anchovy fillets, drained and cut in thirds
Maldon sea salt and freshly ground pepper

FOR THE CROUTONS

3 medium new potatoes
1 tbsp extra-virgin olive oil
2 garlic cloves, finely chopped
1/3 tsp dried Cajun seasoning or 1 tsp fresh (see page 43)
Maldon sea salt
3 tbsp finely grated Parmesan cheese

FOR THE DRESSING

3 medium-sized lemons, juiced
1/4 garlic clove, finely chopped or crushed
4 tbsp extra-virgin olive oil
several dashes of Worcestershire sauce
1 free-range organic egg

HERE'S HOW

To prepare the croutons, first preheat the oven to 220°C/425°F/Gas Mark 7. Spray a non-stick baking sheet with vegetable cooking spray or wipe with olive oil. Wash the potatoes, leaving on the skins, cut them in wedges 15 mm (1/2 in) wide and then again to make cubes. Drain the potato chunks in a colander and spread them out on a double layer of paper towels to dry. Mix together the olive oil, pepper, salt, finely grated Parmesan and Cajun seasoning in a large bowl and drop the potato cubes into it using your fingers to coat them. Add a bit more olive oil if you need it. Bake the potato chunks for 15 to 20 minutes, turning them occasionally so they brown evenly. Remove from the oven and drain on double layers of paper towels to cool.

To prepare the dressing, mix together the lemon juice, garlic, olive oil and Worcestershire sauce in a small bowl. Break the whole egg into the jar and whisk with a fork or whisk to blend well.

Then, for the salad, wash and dry the romaine leaves. Tear the leaves into chunky morsels, wrap them in a clean tea towel and chill in the refrigerator until needed. Place the romaine chunks in a large, flat salad bowl, add the cooled potato croutons and pour the freshly made salad dressing over all. Add the anchovies and season. Toss and serve topped with shaved Parmesan.

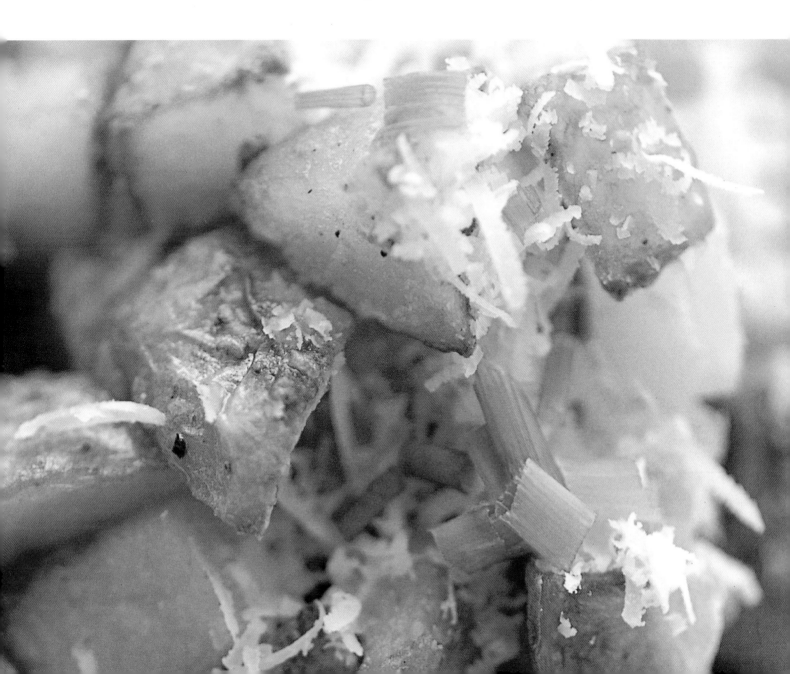

WILD HERB SALAD

The most powerful of all groups of plants for health are the herbs. This is because they tend to be richer than the fruits and vegetables in terms of their antioxidant and other health-giving phytochemicals. But there is something else involved too. Herbs have to struggle hard to survive. This means that any weakness that may have originally appeared in the plant is likely to have been weeded out over a multitude of generations; otherwise the plant would not have survived. Herbs therefore have a very strong life force that they can bring to us.

I use herbs as often as I can in what I cook, and I like to use them raw whenever possible. In fact, when I'm using a herb such as sage, thyme or rosemary in a cooked dish I often cook what needs to be cooked and then add the herb right at the end. In this way it maintains all its wonderful nutritional and energetic properties - not to mention its brighter colour and stronger taste.

My favourite way of eating herbs - above all else - is in a wild herb salad. This is a salad you can make with almost anything. But the more wild herbs you use, and the more dark green vegetables, the better it works. Even the flavour of this salad is wild. Its nutritional value is superb.

To make this salad (see the recipe overleaf) you certainly don't need all the ingredients listed here. You can make it with as little as two or three different herbs. I love to sprinkle the whole lot afterwards with edible flowers, like marigold petals, just for colour. This is a recipe that you can make a hundred ways and it works out perfectly each time. Don't be afraid to omit ingredients such as olives or lovage if you don't happen to have any. Just one word of warning - when it comes to choosing your light green lettuce, don't go for iceberg since the flavour does not work with herbs, but you can use chicory. The salad needs little tossing. Some of its ingredients are very strong, but others are rather fragile, so what it does need is careful handling.

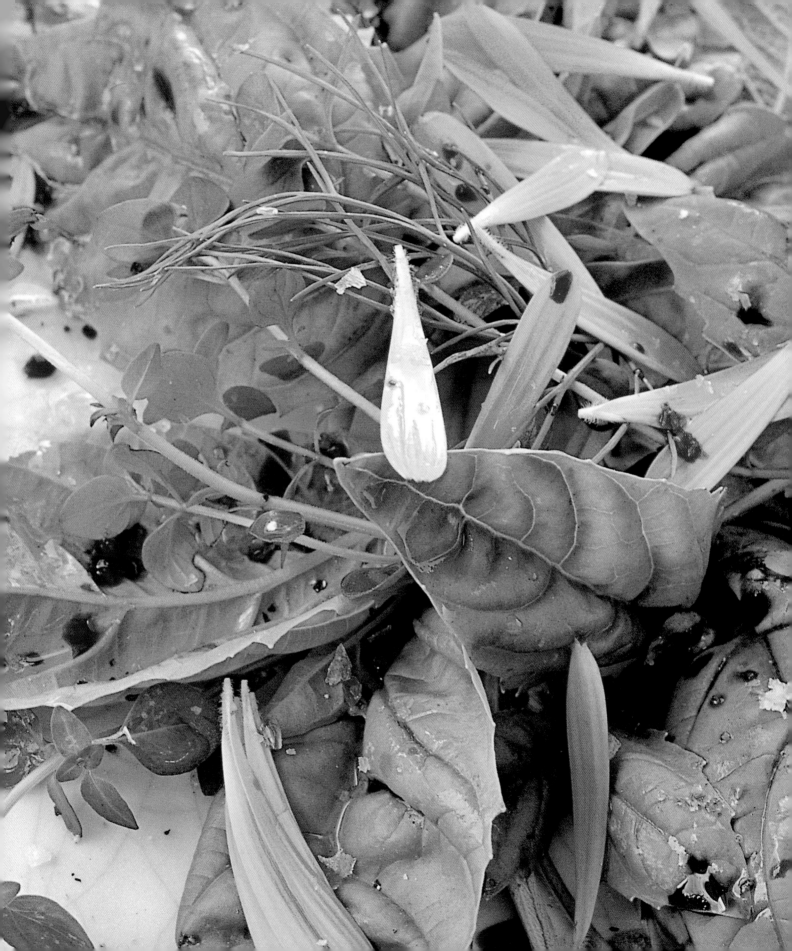

WHAT YOU NEED FOR THE SALAD

1 large bunch fresh organic
   rocket or 2 hearts cos
   lettuce, sliced or torn
1 light green lettuce
18 sprigs of lamb's lettuce
12 leaves of purslane
18 leaves of fresh basil
1 small bunch of fresh tarragon
6 sprigs of lovage
12 leaves of broad-leaf parsley
1 small radicchio
1 red onion, chopped, or some
   fat red radishes, slivered
1 yellow pepper, sliced
1 red pepper, sliced
handful of fat black olives
handful of marigold petals
a few sprigs of fennel
mint leaves (optional)

FOR THE DRESSING

6 tbsp extra-virgin olive oil
3 tbsp balsamic vinegar
several dashes of
   Worcestershire sauce
Maldon sea salt and freshly
   ground pepper
a dash of Cajun seasoning
(see page 43)

HERE'S HOW

Wash the rocket and lettuce and dry in a salad basket, then dry and shred diagonally in medium pieces or tear in bite-size chunks and place in a flat salad bowl. Chill this in the refrigerator for half an hour. Wash the lamb's lettuce, getting rid of the root ends, then whirl it in a salad basket to dry and wrap it in a tea towel to chill. Wash and prepare all the other ingredients similarly and chill them for 15 minutes.

When you are ready to serve the salad, remove the salad bowl from the refrigerator. Arrange the herbs and sprigs, including the lamb's lettuce, in the bowl and add whatever additions, such as peppers, red peppers, radishes or olives, that you wish. Now add the dressing ingredients one by one on top of the salad and toss lightly. Garnish with flower petals, fennel and mint if you happen to have it, and serve on individual flat dishes.

BRIGHTER THE BETTER

When it comes to Crunchy Feasts, whatever recipe you're making it's worth remembering the old saying that an apple a day keeps the doctor away. These days, the apple has been replaced by several portions of bright-coloured vegetables. And there is no better way of eating them than in a fresh and crunchy bright-coloured salad. From red peppers and carrots to beetroot, marrows, rocket, cabbages and Swiss chard – even sweet potatoes and pumpkins – the vegetables in the red/orange/yellow family are rich in carotenoids and other phytonutrients such as the flavonoids. The beneficial effects of the carotenoids in brightly coloured fruits and vegetables are given below. (For the Inside Story on carotenoids, see page 86.)

* Carotenoids carry anti-tumour activity, helping to protect us from cancer and probably from many other degenerative illnesses as well, such as ageing skin. Carotenoids are not the only phytochemicals that help protect against degeneration. So do the phenols and ellagic acid. Fibre in vegetables is important too.

* Carotenoids act in the human body very much as they do in plant cells from which they come. They offer protection as a cellular screen against photo-oxidative damage, from the sun as well as other kinds of free-radical damage.

* A high intake of both beta-carotene and the other carotenoids is associated with a significantly reduced rate of skin cancer, lung cancer and cervical cancer, probably because beta-carotene helps improve the integrity of the epithelial cells.

* Carotenoids also help prevent heart disease. In one study, carried out over a 13-year period, scientists discovered that there is a very strong correlation between low concentrations of carotenoids in the blood and increased heart disease.

ONE-BOWL MEALS

4

I love one-bowl eating. Maybe it is an atavistic regression to my peasant ancestors, but the idea of sitting down to a big .bowl of fish soup or Dhal stew, seems great fun. Best of all are the one-bowl salads, which come complete with good quality protein – tofu, prawns or chicken. The single most important change you can make to your diet for energy and good looks is to make one meal a day a one-bowl salad. In two weeks you look and feel like a new person. One-bowls in any form consist of colourful, simple, tasty food which is as good for you as it is delicious, makes a meal that is a pleasure to eat alone or share with others. The trouble is, once you get into creating one-bowl meals, you can begin to wonder

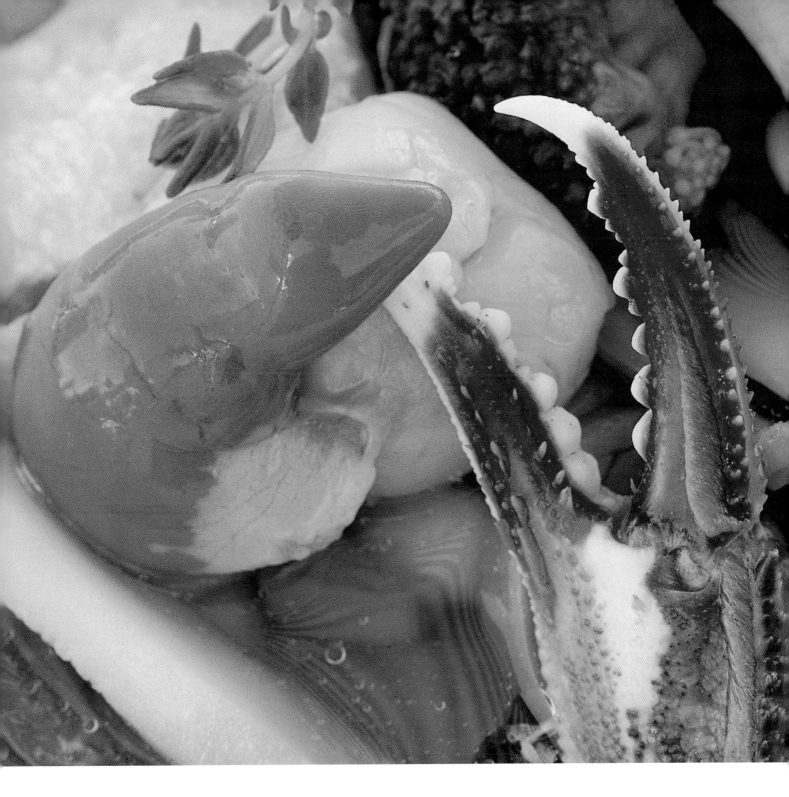

WHY YOU EVER DID **ANYTHING ELSE.**

GO FISH

Just about everybody these days knows that fish - and now shellfish - is supposed to be good for you. The hullabaloo about fish began when researchers discovered that the Eskimos, who traditionally lived on a very high fat diet based on fish and seafood, had stunningly low rates of heart disease and cancer. So impressive was this research - most of it done in the mid-eighties - that a diet which revolves around fish and seafood as the primary source of protein and fat has become almost a fad ever since. Yet it is a fad with a purpose. It is quite true that a diet high in fish protects against many degenerative diseases from gallstones and colitis to arthritis, diabetes, heart disease and cancer. (For the Inside Story on fish, see page 92.)

serves 6

LA BOURRIDE PACIFICA

I like this one-bowl meal so much that I could quite literally live on it; the photograph for this recipe is shown on the previous page. It is easy to make and completely adaptable to whatever fish you can find. Because I adore the fish you get in the Southern Hemisphere - especially the wide variety and the unbeatable freshness - this recipe calls for a number of fishes available in the South Pacific. The truth is you can use just about any kind of seafood to make this wonderful meal.

Another thing I like about this fish soup is that it is so cheap to make. Go to your fishmonger or supermarket and ask them for all the parts of fresh fish they usually throw away - the skeletons, the heads, the fins. Toss them all into a pot and make the fish stock (see page 178). This you can keep in the refrigerator for two to three days or in the freezer for two to three months. You will use this not only for La bourride Pacifica but any number of other dishes. If you are feeling really lazy go and buy fish sauce, which you will find in any Oriental shop or in the speciality section of a good supermarket, and mix it with water to make the stock. But it is so much more delicious to make your own stock, and fun too.

For the fish in this recipe try to mix fish and shellfish so you end up with large pieces of fish, some clams or mussels, some shellfish and some small pieces of fish or even tiny whole fish. The more variety you get, the more gorgeous will be the result. Look for variety in colour too. Here are some of my favourites, but go for whatever is cheap and easy to come by: snapper, cod, groper, turbot, bass, salmon, eel, halibut, mussels, clams, prawns.

WHAT YOU NEED

4 carrots, cut into julienne strips
2 leeks, just the white parts, chopped in ringlets
1 fennel bulb, chopped
100 g (4 oz) chopped broccoli
100 g (4 oz) spring onions, sliced
1 tbsp extra-virgin olive oil
1.5 litres (2 1/2 pints) fish stock
500 ml (18 fl oz) dry white wine
1.5 kg (3 lb 7 oz) of 5 to 8 varieties of fish and shellfish
2 tsp roughly cut lemon zest
lemon grass

HERE'S HOW

Sear the vegetables briefly in olive oil. Do not cook clear through. Bring the fish stock and the wine to the boil. Toss the vegetables into the stock and add the largest pieces of fish and shellfish. A minute later add the medium pieces. A minute later, add the tiny fishes, clams and mussels. Cook for another couple of minutes and serve immediately with Aïoli or Aïoli Lite on the side **(see pages 178 and 179)** and bread.

serves 4 generously

GRILLED PRAWNS AND ROCKET SALAD

There is some magic about grilled prawns and rocket mixed together - I've no idea why. I've tried to figure it out more than once. All I know is that the richness of prawns and the crunchiness of rocket - especially if you can get wild rocket - is worth any amount of effort to get together. The lovely thing about this salad is that it's no effort to make. You can grill the prawns ahead of time and simply take them out of the refrigerator and add to the rocket, or you can grill them, as I tend to do, on a teppan yaki grill and serve them immediately on top of the rocket.

WHAT YOU NEED
400 g (14 oz) tiger prawns
2 tbsp extra-virgin olive oil
100 g (4 oz) rocket, washed
    and with any heavy stems
    removed
2 garlic cloves, chopped
zest and juice of 1/2 a lemon
Maldon sea salt and freshly
    ground red or black
    peppercorns

HERE'S HOW
Peel the prawns and run a knife down their backs to pull away any small black threads. Rinse and pat dry. Heat the pan or grill, coating with a little olive oil. Cook the prawns quickly at a high temperature for about 3 minutes until they start to go golden. While they're cooking, sprinkle them with the garlic, lemon zest, Maldon sea salt and coarsely ground pepper.

Line a flat salad bowl with the rocket. The moment the prawns are done, remove from the heat. Add a garlicky-vinaigrette dressing to the rocket, place the prawns on top, sprinkle with lemon juice and coarsely ground black or red peppercorns and serve immediately.

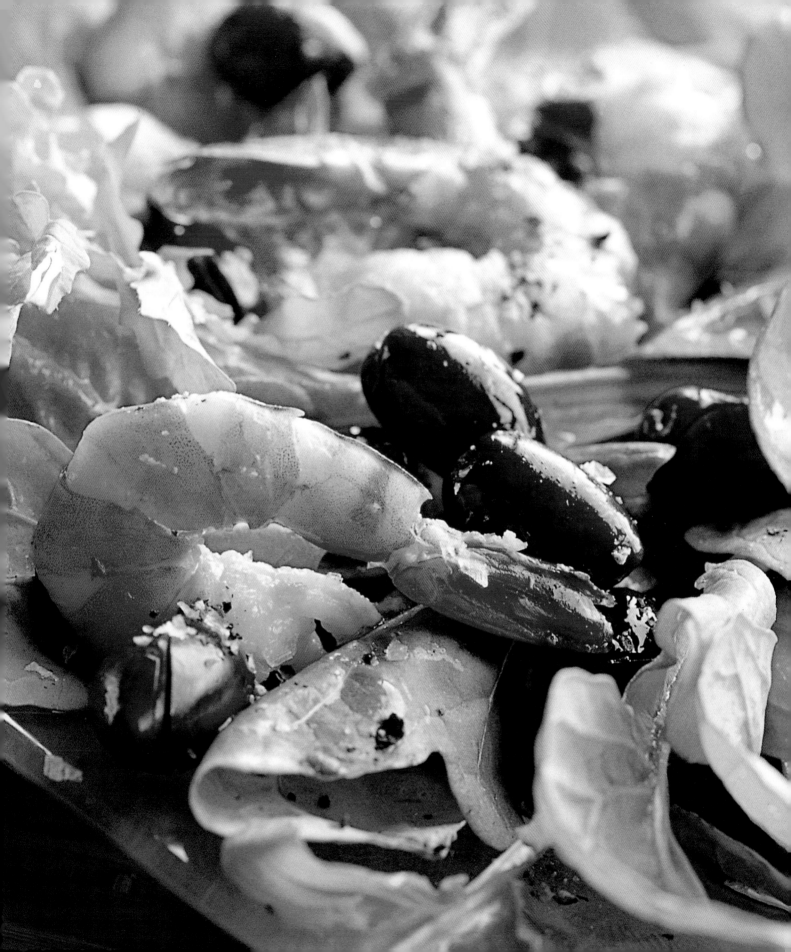

MUSSELS STRAIGHT UP

Mussels are my favourite shellfish. Whatever mussels you buy make sure they come from unpolluted waters and are alive. If you think they are likely to be sandy then soak them overnight in a bucket of water to which you have added a couple of tablespoons of cornflour. The mussels will feed on the cornflour and in return expel any sand they have collected. (For the Inside Story on mussels, see page 92.)

WHAT YOU NEED

2 kg (4 lb 8 oz) green-lipped mussels
6 tbsp extra-virgin olive oil
1 large onion, finely chopped
3 garlic cloves, finely chopped
250 ml (8 fl oz) dry white wine
2.5 cm (1 in) piece of fresh ginger, finely shredded
small handful of arami seaweed (soak for 1 to 2 hours and then drain) (optional)
zest of 1 lemon, finely shredded
Maldon sea salt and freshly ground pepper
2 red peppers, roughly chopped
small bunch of fresh basil, chopped
small bunch of fresh flat-leaved parsley, chopped
2 green chillies, finely chopped

HERE'S HOW

Scrub the outer shells of the mussels with a stiff brush in cold water and pull out the beards that stick to the sides. Throw away any mussels with broken shells and any that remain open when you are handling them. In a large pot heat the olive oil and gently fry the onion and garlic for 5 minutes, stirring regularly. Add the wine, ginger, arami (if using), lemon zest and seasoning and bring to the boil. Toss in the mussels and cover, steaming them for 2 to 3 minutes until the shells open.

Discard any that have remained shut after cooking. Now tuck the remaining ingredients into the open shells with your fingers to garnish. The contrast between the colours of the garnishes and the sea-earth shades of the mussels is one of the great pleasures of making this dish. Serve immediately in the sauce.

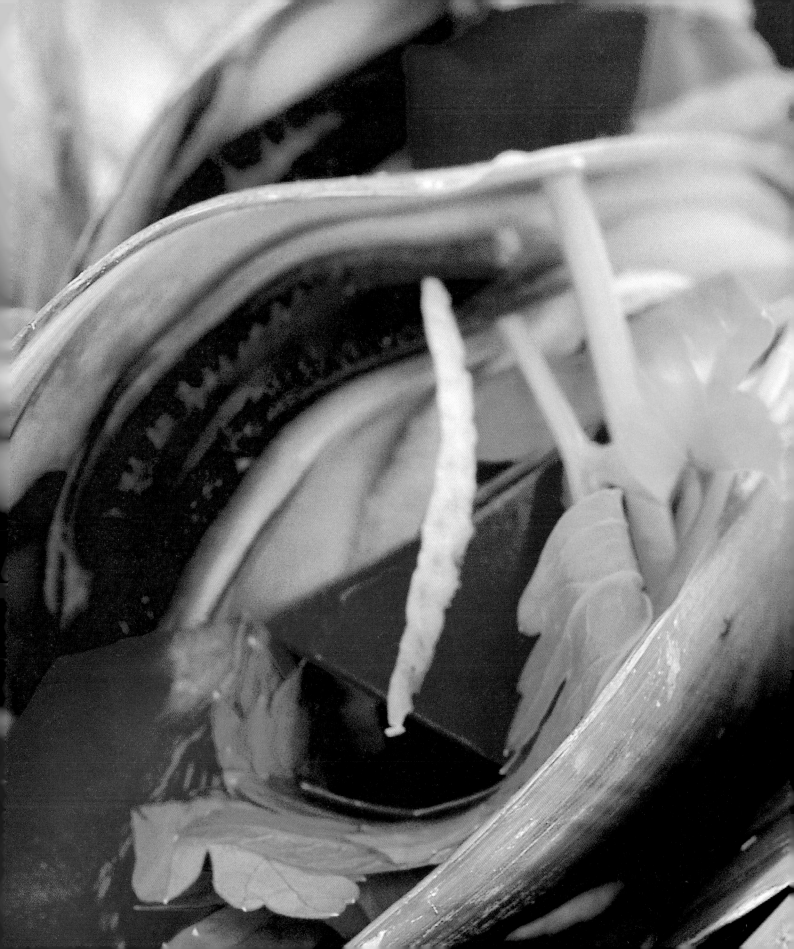

BEANS, SEEDS AND GRAINS

The heroic virtues of beans – from adzuki and black-eyed peas to chickpeas, kidney beans, fava, lentils, soya, navy beans and split peas – has been much touted in recent years in relation to what they can do for health. This may be why our consumption of beans and legumes has increased almost 50 percent in the last ten years.

Protective powers

A number of studies show that pulses help prevent cancer and heart disease. They also help stabilize blood-sugar levels and even counter obesity. These legumes are rich in both soluble and insoluble fibre – so rich that 175 g (6 oz) of lentils contains as much fibre as five large potatoes – in effect, half of the daily recommendation of 30 g (just over 1 oz). A recent research project at Oxford University confirmed that a legume-rich diet helps control diabetes by lowering blood-sugar levels and improves the quality of blood fats. Pulses are also rich in lignans – phyto-oestrogens – to help regulate hormonal balance in the body. They offer too some protection against many kinds of cancer including breast cancer. Legumes are low in fat, low in sodium and high in protein, particularly when they are eaten together with wholegrain breads, so that you get a full complement of both essential and non-essential amino acids from which your body can build new protein.

For the vegetarian, beans and legumes are musts. The problem is that many people find pulses difficult to digest. They are known for their ability to produce flatulence and they make some people feel heavy – all of which goes to show that no matter how good something is for you, too much is not so good. I like to use legumes either in whole meal soups and stews or to take them and make filling yet low-fat dips by mixing them with a little olive oil, some fresh herbs and seasoning.

serves 6

DHAL STEW

I make this either with red lentils or dried yellow split peas. It has a curry flavour and is full of coarsely chopped vegetables. (For the Inside Story on onions, see page 88.)

WHAT YOU NEED

250 g (9 oz) red lentils or
    split peas
720 ml (1 1/4 pints) stock or
    2 tbsp of low-fat vegetable
    bouillon powder plus 720 ml
    (1 1/4 pints) water
1 large onion, finely chopped
5 garlic cloves, coarsely
    chopped
1/2 tsp turmeric
pinch of ginger
1 large cauliflower, broken
    into florets
3 large carrots, roughly
    chopped
1 large parsnip, roughly
    chopped
100 g (4 oz) broccoli florets
2 large tomatoes, chopped, or
    3 tbsp of tomato paste plus
    125 ml (4 fl oz) water
1 red pepper, chopped
1 yellow pepper, chopped
2 tsp ground cumin
1 bunch of fresh coriander,
    coarsely chopped
1-2 tbsp mild curry powder
Maldon sea salt and freshly
    ground pepper

HERE'S HOW

Put the red lentils or split peas into a large pot and cover with stock, or use 720 ml (1 1/4 pints) and 1 tablespoon of low-fat vegetable bouillon powder. Cook for 45 minutes until tender. Purée in a food processor and set aside. While they are cooking, braise the onion in a little water with the garlic, turmeric, ginger and 1 tablespoon vegetable bouillon powder. When they have softened, add all the vegetables and the other seasonings and simmer until cooked. Pour the puréed legume mixture into the vegetables, mix to heat through and serve immediately.

SPROUT SALAD

Eat sprout salads often. It can change your life. Seeds and grains are latent powerhouses of nutritional goodness and life energy. They are plants at the point of greatest vitality. When you sprout and eat them, this vitality gets transmitted to you.

Most seeds and grains are cheap and readily available in supermarkets or health food stores - chickpeas, brown lentils, mung beans, wheat grains and so forth. Since you can sprout them yourself with nothing but clean water, they become an easily accessible source of organically grown fresh vegetables, even for city dwellers. In an age when most vegetables and fruits are grown on artificially fertilized soils and treated with hormones, fungicides, insecticides, preservatives and all manner of other chemicals, the home-grown-in-a-jar sprouts emerge as a pristine blessing - fresh, unpolluted and ready to eat in a minute by popping them into salads or sandwiches. Seeds can be a lot of fun to sprout too **(see page 183 for how to sprout your own seeds)**.

The trick to making a great sprout salad is to mix these light-as-air vegetables with something richer and creamier such as a good mayonnaise or avocado dressing and then spike them with something larger and crunchier - say chicory or julienned carrots or even apples. **(For the Inside Story on sprouts, see page 89.)**

WHAT YOU NEED
50 g (2 oz) mangetout sprouts
25 g (1 oz) radish or mustard
  sprouts
50 g (2 oz) alfalfa sprouts
1/2 chicory or other lettuce in
  large pieces
1/2 bunch of watercress
8 slices of teppan yaki-grilled
  tofu **(see page 136)**
a few fresh edible flowers
  (optional)

HERE'S HOW
Wash and dry the sprouts and wrap in a tea towel. Place in the refrigerator for 15 minutes or more to crisp up while you prepare the other ingredients. Then place everything but the tofu in a bowl, pour a garlicky vinaigrette **(see page 184)** over the raw vegetables and toss gently. Add the tofu slices on top and serve immediately decorated with an edible flower or two if you have them in the garden.

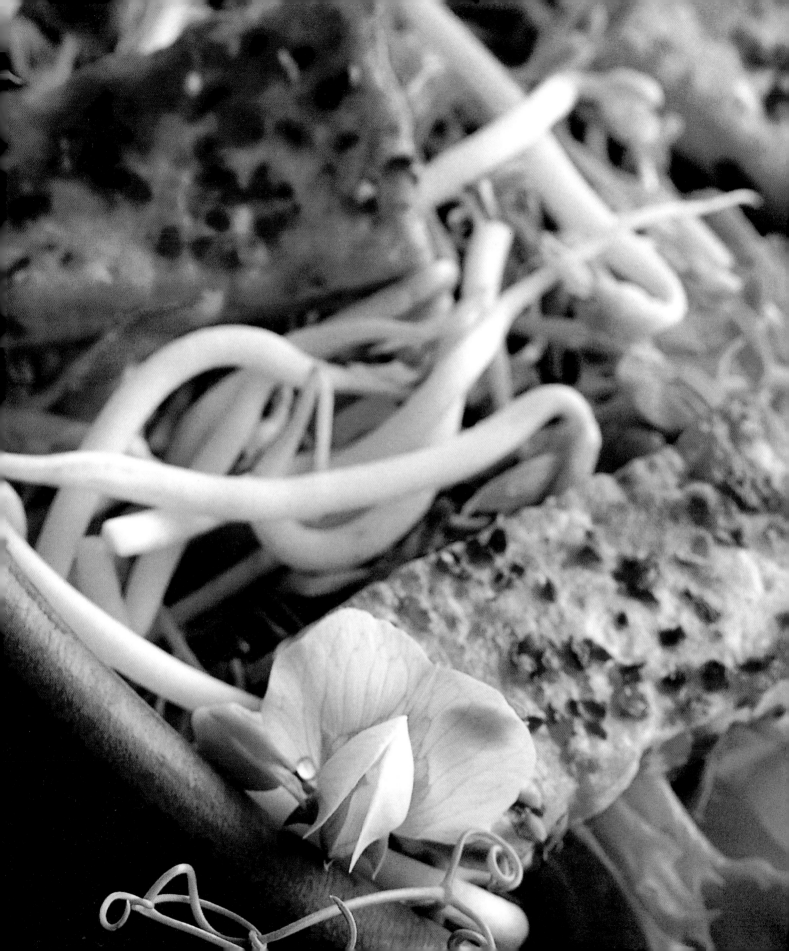

ON THE MOVE

5

I like to make every meal a picnic - an adventure. I try to keep from falling into habits with food either by eating the same thing over and over or by eating in the same place with the same plates. If the sun is shining on the landing then take a tablecloth and eat there. Eat in bed. Sit on your children's beds and have lunch with them when they are ill. Eat as often as you can in the open air. When you travel, take a simple but beautifully packed meal with you on the train or plane.

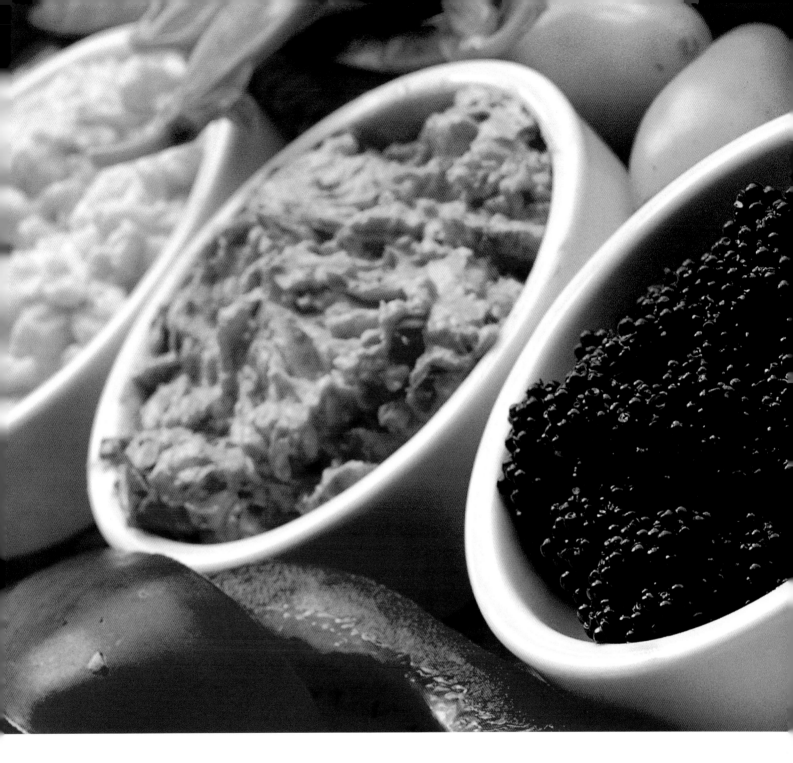

MAKE IT A HAPPENING.

ENERGY BITES

There is no more delicious way to reap the benefits of energy-enhancing vegetables than munching on a platter of crudités: crunchy raw vegetables sliced or slivered and garnished with lemon slices, sprigs of watercress or fresh basil and served with rich and wonderful dipping sauces. Whether you tuck them into a lunch box or serve them on a wooden platter in the garden or in bed, these finger foods make ideal on-the-go eating.

Anything goes

Most crudités fall short of their potential because people get stuck in a rut when preparing them. For crudités to work you need real variety – not only in the sauces you serve with them but also in the raw materials themselves. Use a mandolin to make chunky chips of carrots, turnips, courgettes and celery. Serve them with knife-sliced hunks of green peppers and red peppers. Don't forget the bigger foods too. Whole leaves of chicory and bok choy torn from the plant, washed and crisped up are great dipped into tapenades or into a mixture of chopped hard-boiled eggs, lean mayonnaise and Cajun seasoning.

Crudités don't have to be all-raw either. An artichoke steamed and chilled makes a wonderful dunking partner, as do blanched florets of broccoli or cauliflower. You can create a good selection of crudités from almost anything you happen to have in the refrigerator. Some of my favourites are young spring onions, button mushrooms, mangetout, which have been topped and tailed, cherry tomatoes, radishes, cucumber in big chunks, kohl rabi and small beetroots. Even slices of apple or pineapple make a nice addition. I like to wash my vegetables and cut or tear or slice them, giving as much variety as possible to the combinations, then dip them in ice water and put them in the refrigerator for half an hour before draining and serving. Lemon juice squeezed atop the drained and dried vegetables keeps them fresh. Always offer a great variety of dipping sauces.

FISH SANDWICH

As a kid I was in love with tuna sandwiches on rye. I ate so many that at one point I was even munching on them for breakfast. Because of the mercury build-up that can take place in you when you indulge in such a practice, it finally occurred to me there might be a better way. Here it is - a fish sandwich that is simple to make, travels well and is much more delicious than canned fish. I grill a piece of boneless fish such as tuna, sword fish, or moon fish or even thin-sliced cod on a teppan yaki grill (see page 136). Then I make an open-faced sandwich using whatever dipping sauces I happen to have or just some plain mayonnaise. I like to add fresh tomatoes and lots of sprouts. If the fish is pre-cooked it takes only a couple of minutes to make for a quick movable feast.

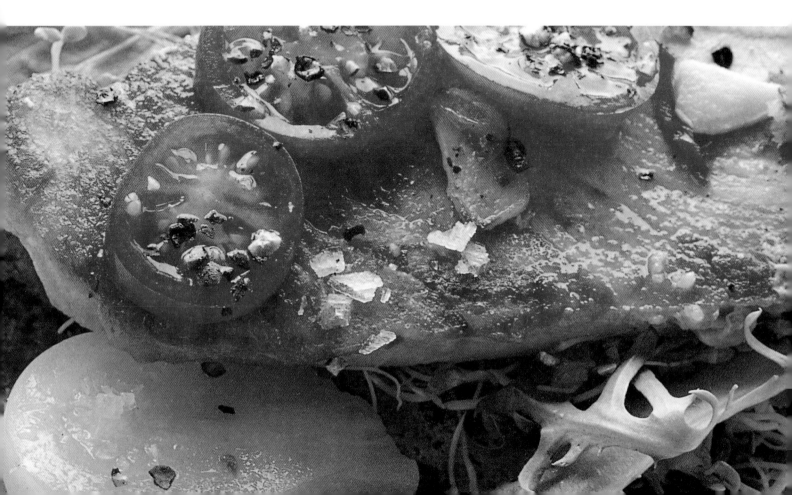

SOBA IN A BOX

serves 2

Long before Americans got into fast food, the Japanese had it worked out. They are masters of convenience foods. Some of the lunch-to-go recipes you find on the streets of Osaka or Tokyo are the best in the world. The difference between their foods and ours is that many of their processed foods - like kudzu, organic tamari and miso - are naturally processed through fermentation and preparations that have been carried out for centuries. As a result, much of their packaged food is actually good for you.

Buckwheat soba is such a food. It is made from the edible fruit seed of the buckwheat plant, which comes originally from the Orient and is a relative of rhubarb - not at all a grain as many people assume. It is a hearty food high in protein and potassium as well as B complex vitamins, calcium, iron and fibre. You can buy buckwheat soba in any Japanese grocers and most good health food stores. They come in two forms: soba, which is 100 percent buckwheat and contains no wheat flour, and the more common, soba noodles, made from a combination of both. I strongly prefer the former. Cook the buckwheat noodles, then serve hot or cold. They travel well and are yummy to eat as a lunch or snack any time.

WHAT YOU NEED
200 g (7 oz) soba noodles
2 carrots, finely slivered (optional)
2 garlic cloves, finely chopped
5 cm (2 in) piece of fresh ginger, finely slivered
2 tbsp spring onions, finely chopped
125 ml (4 fl oz) mirin, white wine or water
a few drops of sesame oil
3 tsp tamari
1 small red pepper, finely chopped

HERE'S HOW
Bring a saucepan filled with water to a rolling boil. Put in the carrots and soba noodles and follow the manufacturer's instructions to cook. When finished, remove from the heat and rinse under cold water in a colander. Meanwhile, sauté the garlic, ginger and spring onions in the mirin, wine or water in a heavy pan for 5 to 7 minutes so that some of the liquid evaporates. Now add the sesame oil, tamari and red pepper, mix and remove from heat. Pour the sautéed mixture over the cooled soba.

Seaweed dipping sauce

Because I so love dipping sauces, I make this seaweed-based one
to go with my soba noodles when I choose to serve them hot. It is
easy to make, so delicious and so good for hair and nails, not to
mention overall metabolism thanks to seaweed's mineral content. I
make a seaweed stock by soaking several pieces of kombu - kelp
leaves - in 375 ml (12 fl oz) of spring water overnight. Then I
simmer this stock for a very few minutes adding 4 tablespoons of
tamari, 4 tablespoons of mirin, 1 tablespoon of honey and a pinch
of salt. I add some chopped spring onions and sesame seeds at the
last minute and dip.

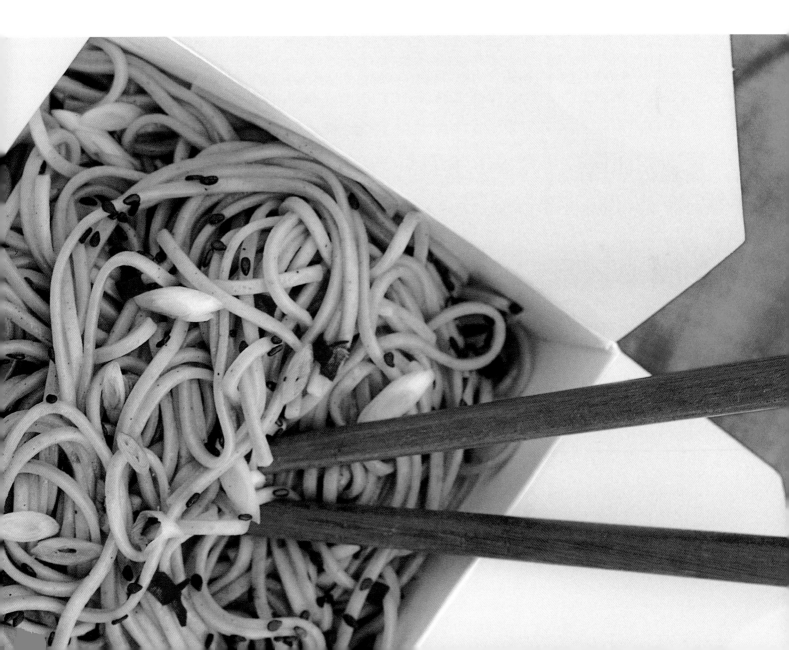

GIFTS FROM THE SEA

The power of sea vegetables for creating high-level well being and strengthening the body is unparalleled in the plant kingdom. Perhaps this is because, biologically as well as mythologically, the sea is said to be the source out of which all life has come. Our blood contains more than a hundred minerals and trace elements found equally in the sea and in the plants that live there. Sea plants contain up to twenty times the minerals of land plants plus a great abundance of vitamins and other phytochemicals that are useful for health. Much of the fibre in seaweeds is so powerful in its ability to help the body detoxify that it can even remove radioactive and toxic metals. (For the Inside Story on seaweeds, see page 93.)

SEAWEED SALADS

serves 4

Some of my favourite salads are made from seaweed. These salads are so unusual in look and flavour that most people would never think to make them. The key to making a beautiful one is to use more than one kind of seaweed. Hijiki is one I use frequently. I also like wakame and arami. You can, however, use some of the others such as dulce and even nori, although when using nori in a salad it's best to toast it very quickly - for 15 to 20 seconds under a grill or in a frying pan. Then break it up in small pieces and sprinkle on the top, otherwise it tends to go soggy.

WHAT YOU NEED
150 g (5 oz) dried seaweeds
1 light-coloured lettuce, e.g. curly endive, little gem, iceberg (shredded), chicory
2 large carrots, julienned
3 small turnips, julienned
40 g (1 1/2 oz) sesame seeds

FOR THE DRESSING
1 tbsp cold pressed sesame oil or Udo's Choice **(see Resources)**
2 tbsp umeboshi vinegar, rice vinegar or lemon juice
2 shallots, finely chopped
2 garlic cloves, chopped
Maldon sea salt and freshly ground pepper

HERE'S HOW

Soak the seaweeds for 30 minutes in water and then drain. Wash the lettuce and then chill both for 15 minutes if possible, since this salad is more delicious chilled than at room temperature. You can serve it at room temperature as well, which is one of the reasons why this salad makes such an excellent picnic food. Unlike most salads it does not go limp, especially if you choose a good, crisp, light-coloured lettuce. Line your salad bowl with the lettuce, then, after draining the seaweeds, add the julienned carrots and turnips.

Now place all the dressing ingredients in a jar and shake well. Pour over the seaweed, carrot and turnip mixture and toss. Arrange this on the bed of lettuce (I do not put dressing on the lettuce because this prevents the lettuce from going limp and is particularly important if you are going to use this salad for a picnic.) Now toast the seasame seeds on an oil-free frying pan or under the grill and sprinkle over everything immediately before serving.

This salad will keep in good condition for several hours if you want to take it on a picnic.

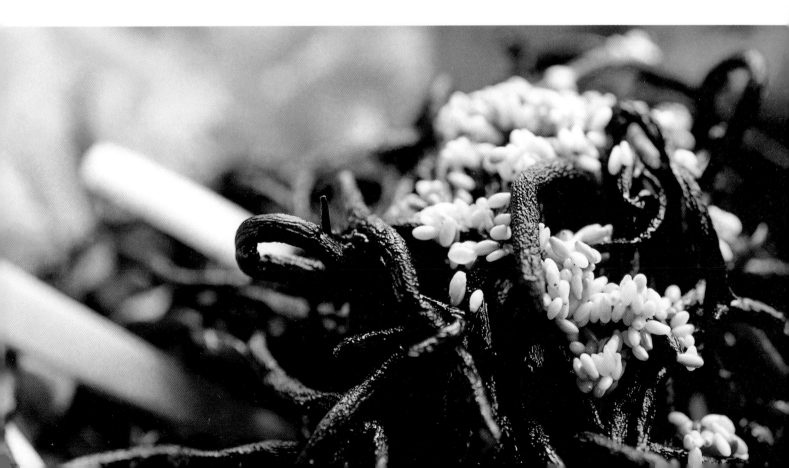

CHUNKY POTATO SALAD

I've always loved potato salad, but I cannot stand the mushy, squared-off variety. I prefer to make mine not with mayonnaise but with a very light dressing – one that is just enough to cover the potatoes with seasoning or herbs and help maintain their integrity. My favourite dressings for this potato salad are Olive Oil, Basil and Lemon Dressing and Wholegrain Mustard and Garlic Dressing, which are given on **page 184**.

WHAT YOU NEED

500 g (1 lb 2 oz) potatoes
handful of mangetout tendrils
    (optional)
a light dressing **(see page 184)**
Maldon sea salt and freshly
    ground pepper

HERE'S HOW

Scrub the potatoes and cook them in salted boiling water just enough that they fall off the blade of a knife or fork when you stick it in. Never cook them until they get mushy. As soon as they're cooked, remove from the heat, drain and put into a bowl. It is at this point that you want to add the mangetout tendrils and the dressing, so that the potatoes absorb it. I often serve my potato salad steaming hot, but it is equally delicious cold.

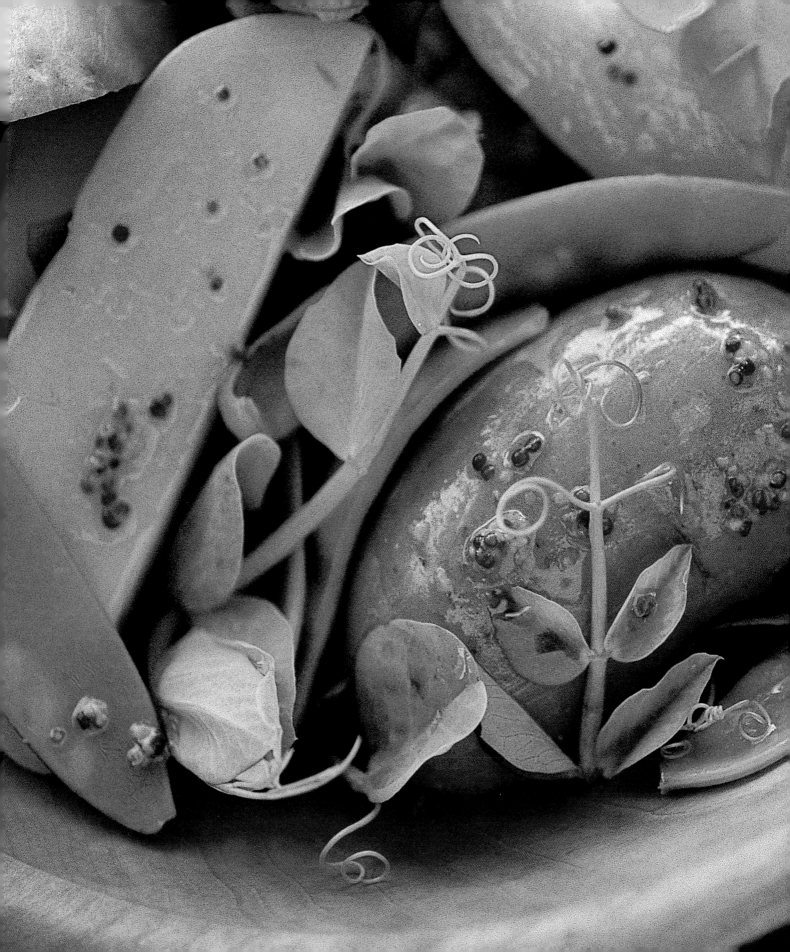

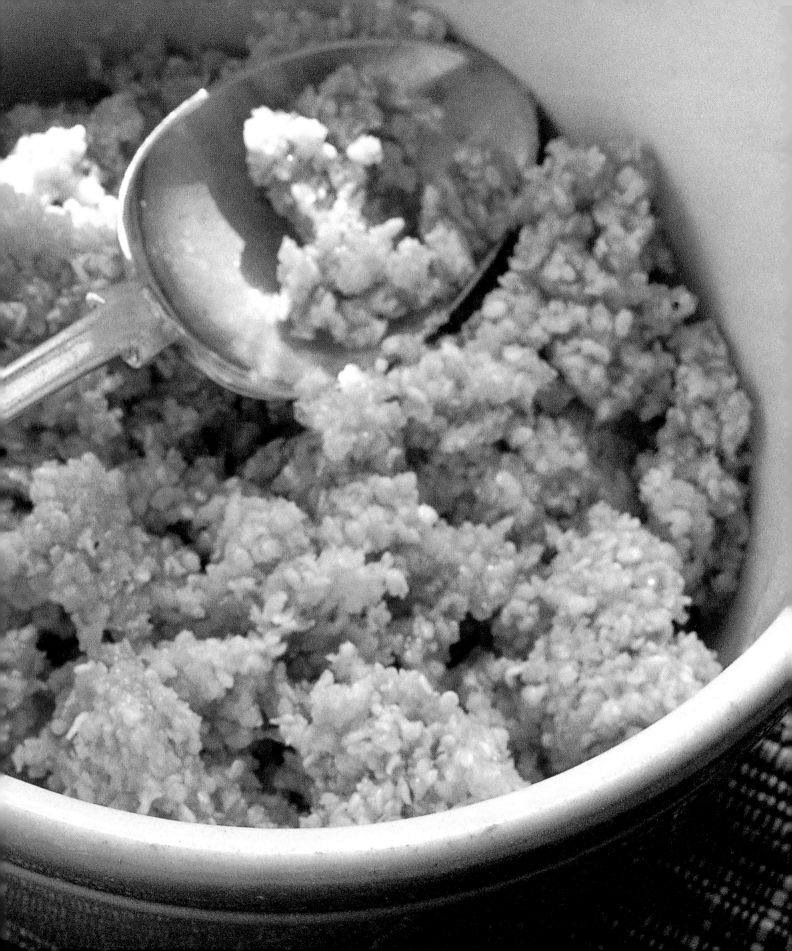

makes 12-36

ROSE MACAROONS

This is my ultra-feminine version of the wonderful amaretto cookies from Italy. It uses pure rosewater - an ingredient I often add to sauces and vinegars - I even make a rosewater chicken. These are delicious little sweets to carry with you wherever you go. When it comes to grinding the almonds used in this recipe, I like to use a coffee grinder to do this as it's instantaneous and turns them into a fine powder.

WHAT YOU NEED
4 egg whites
300 g (10 oz) golden granulated sugar
300 g (10 oz) almonds, finely ground
3 tsp rosewater
2 tbsp finely grated fresh or dried coconut

HERE'S HOW
Preheat the oven to 170°C/325°F/Gas Mark 3. Whisk the egg whites until stiff. Now add half the sugar and gently combine. Then mix in the other half and fold in the ground almonds. Sprinkle on the rosewater and gently fold it in too. Drop teaspoonfuls of the mixture on baking trays that have been lined with greaseproof paper and bake for 20 to 30 minutes until golden-brown. Allow them to cool for 5 minutes on the trays. Then gently sprinkle the little cookies with more rosewater and dust the top with finely grated coconut.

THE INSIDE STORY

By now you've experienced a little of the Cook Energy way of eating for power, and know how much fun it can be, here is some more in-depth information on just what these fabulous foods can do for you. For decades the study of the relationship between food and health has consisted of amassing information about how many vitamins and minerals, how much protein and carbohydrate and what kind of essential fatty acids we need to stay healthy. For too long, popular nutrition focused on urging that we take high-potency, man-made nutritional supplements. Predictions were that by the year 2000 we would all be taking pills instead of bothering with making meals. When it came to the meals we do eat, we were told mostly about what we shouldn't eat too much of. Lower your sugar and saturated fats intake. Eat less meat – and so on. Forget it. Now is the time to

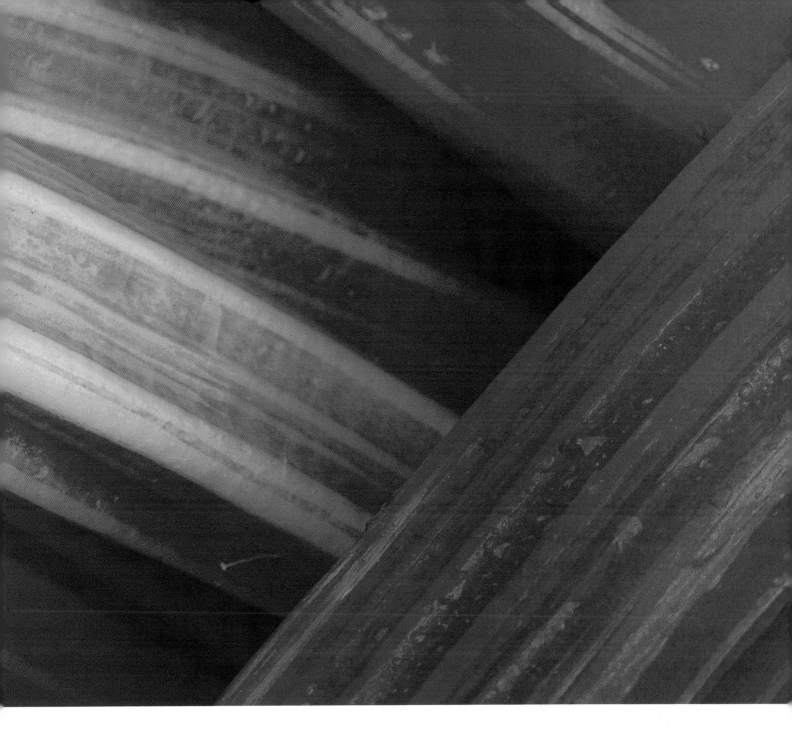

EAT MORE

AND THRIVE.

Nutritionists are increasingly aware that vitamins and minerals, essential fatty acids, proteins, carbohydrates and sugars are only a very small part of eating for high-level health. The latest research indicates that there is no way we can take vitamin and mineral supplements yet continue to eat highly processed foods and still stay healthy. Why? Because the ability of food to enhance health and beauty is finally being recognized. Not only does enough vitamin C prevent scurvy and enough calcium and magnesium help build strong bones; foods also contain important phytochemicals. These are plant-based substances and compounds that have specific effects on the body. The only way to reap their benefits is to eat whole foods. Second – also as a result of this recent research – the focus of eating for health is no longer on eating less of this or that; it is about eating more. More what? More delicious food. And the foods that we are being encouraged to eat more of are wonderful fresh vegetables, fresh fruits, nuts and seeds, whole foods and grains, fish, organic poultry and organic meat.

FUTURE NUTRITION

The nutritional revolution has brought with it a brand new vocabulary with words like nutraceuticals, phytochemicals and zoochemicals, which are important to know about. Nutraceuticals (sometimes spelled nutriceuticals) are compounds that have specific health benefits. Within the range of nutraceuticals you will find phytochemicals or phytonutrients. These, in turn, are substances or compounds that we do not produce in our own bodies, but which are available to us when we eat plants – especially in a fresh, preferably raw, state. They have protective and health-enhancing effects on the body. Zoochemicals were first discussed by Antony Almada, a nutritional biochemist. He used the word to describe compounds in fish, dairy products, eggs, meat and poultry that are particularly health enhancing to the human body.

It has only been in the last two or three decades that researchers have begun to explore and identify in detail the bioactive compounds in foods which have antioxidant, anti-cancer and anti-ageing properties. They are able to enhance the immune function, to strengthen various organs, even lower excessive blood pressure and cholesterol. The list of functions that the new nutraceuticals in foods can improve is a very long one indeed, and can only be touched on here.

In addition to the zoochemicals and the phytochemicals there is one more term which is very important to the food-for-health revolution, and that is functional foods. Functional foods have specific health benefits and medicinal properties, and these have generally been well backed up by research. Take garlic, for instance. Garlic is rich in organosulphur compounds. These phytochemicals lower cholesterol levels, reduce blood clotting and lower blood pressure. Soya beans contain protease inhibitors as well as phytic acid, which helps lower cholesterol levels and also protects from cancer. They may even slow the growth of cancerous cells in an organism that already has the illness. Broccoli is rich in indoles and in a substance called sulphoranphane. They help prevent breast cancer.

So powerful are the health-enhancing properties of some phytochemicals found in natural foods that even the United States Food and Drug Administration – the FDA, a highly conservative and rather industry-supporting government body – has come out in favour of their consumption. The FDA now insists that edible fruits and vegetables 'exhibit a potential for modulating human metabolism in a manner favourable for cancer prevention'. As anyone worth their salt in nutrition and biochemistry will tell you, whatever helps prevent cancer is also going to help prevent other degenerative diseases – even premature ageing.

But what we can do is take beautifully grown – preferably organic – foods and prepare them in ways that are not only delicious to eat but also rich in the nutraceuticals that enhance health. The age of 'health foods' is at last coming to an end. It is no longer appropriate for us to do as we did in the seventies and eighties – that is, hold our nose and pile in our morning yoghurt with bran, believing that although it may taste disgusting, it's doing us some good. Let's lay to rest forever the notion that for something to be good for you it has to taste revolting. Healthy meals are meals that are not only radiant with colour and form, they are delicious and fun to prepare.

FANTASTIC FRUIT

Instantly edible and perfectly portable, fruit packs a big punch with its store of phytochemical compounds.

BOUNTEOUS BANANAS

If you were looking for an almost perfect fast food, you could not do better than bananas. Bananas have so many things to offer for health that it would be hard to list them all. Some of the most important points are that they relieve both constipation and diarrhoea, reduce the risk of stroke and heart disease, lift spirits, heighten energy and lower blood pressure that is too high.

Bananas are one of the richest sources of potassium, which few of us get enough of these days since convenience foods are practically without it. Potassium helps regulate blood pressure

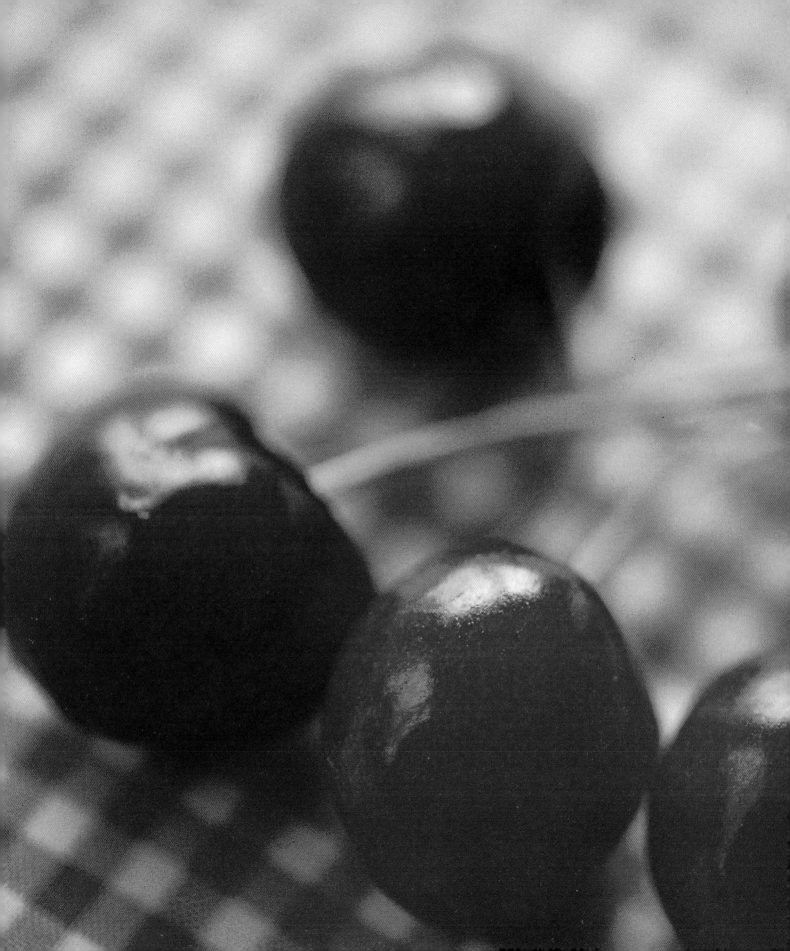

and enhances your body's ability to deal with stress. It also helps get rid of waterlogging, especially in women at the time of a period. And it balances the excessive amounts of sodium many people get from eating highly salted foods. Ripe bananas – especially organic ones – act as natural antacids. In fact, they strengthen the lining of the stomach. Some research shows they may even help kill harmful bacteria in the gut. And they are a great source of pectin – a soluble fibre that helps eliminate harmful chemicals from the body. Always use bananas ripe – never green. If your bananas ripen all at once, peel them and pop into the freezer.

CRUNCH A COCONUT

Coconut is rich in saturated fat but there is some evidence that it is an unusual form of fat with protective properties. I like using fresh coconut whenever possible. I look for heavy coconuts, shake them and listen for lots of liquid. I also check to make sure they have no soft or mouldy spots. You can buy commercially shredded coconut, but lots of food manufacturers add extra sugar to it and propylene glycol to help keep it moist. If you don't have fresh coconut, look for unsweetened shredded or flaked coconut without additives.

CRANBERRIES PROTECT

Cranberries are another of those wonderful red/orange/yellow fruits rich in antioxidants and high in flavour. Native Americans have used them for centuries as a food and as a medicine. They have anti-fungal properties and are anti-viral too, except in the case of Candida albicans, which they don't seem to touch. Cranberries, fresh or dried, help prevent as well as treat urinary infections such as cystitis too. They knock out the *Escherichia coli* bacteria that glue themselves to the walls of the intestine and the bladder. An as yet unidentified phytochemical in cranberries appears to prevent them from sticking. Cranberries also boast a natural antibiotic – hippuric acid. Eating them carries it into the bladder and kidneys.

MANGOES LIFT DEPRESSION

Mangoes have long been called food for the gods. It was Paramahansa Yogananda who wrote in his *Autobiography of a Yogi*, 'It is impossible for the Hindu to conceive of a heaven without mangoes'. He may have known nothing of the biochemistry of this sensuous fruit, but he certainly got right its uplifting properties. Mangoes are rich in anacardic acid and anacardiol – phytochemicals that bear a strong resemblance to the drugs used to treat depression. This makes them a great way to start a day – especially if you can get them tree-ripened and organic.

VEGETABLES FOR VICTORY

Scientists estimate that each of the 60 trillion cells in the human body suffers 10,000 free-radical 'hits' each day. And this is on the increase as a result of increasing chemicals in our environment. Vegetables have powerful antioxidant capacities that help protect against such damage and which go way beyond each vegetable's specfic vitamin and mineral content. The phytonutrients – which give vegetables their distinctive colours and flavours – help to reduce oxidation damage, slowing ageing and degeneration. Already scientists have discovered hundreds of health-enhancing phytochemicals that inhibit blood clotting, lower cholesterol, detoxify the body of wastes and poisons, reduce inflammation and allergies – even slow the growth of cancer cells. These amazing nutraceuticals, most of which were completely unknown ten years ago, work synergistically: the wider the variety of fruits and vegetables you eat, the greater will be the protective health-enhancing benefits for you.

COLOUR YOUR LIFE

Although carotenoids are by no means the only health-enhancing phytochemicals nestled within brightly coloured vegetables, they are probably the most highly researched. These plant pigments, found in the protein complexes of plants, are responsible for many of the bright colours of various fruits and vegetables. You find carotenoids in green plant tissues as well, but in this case they tend to be covered by chlorophyll so thin their presence only becomes evident after the green pigment has degraded as it does when you cook the plant, or when it begins to die in the autumn.

A number of epidemiological studies have shown that the more we eat of fresh fruit and vegetables rich in carotenoids, the more our risk of cancer is diminished. Part of this is due to carotenoids' powerful antioxidant activity. They help protect the body from free-radical damage, which is associated with the development of degenerative conditions from arthritis to coronary heart disease as well as premature ageing. Carotenoids, like some of the vitamins, such as vitamin A, vitamin C and vitamin E, are able to quench free radicals and de-activate them, thereby inhibiting excessive free-radical reactions in our body, and protect us from damage.

Scientists estimate that there are probably more than 600 naturally occurring carotenoids in our foods. They are certainly the most widespread pigments found in nature. The most well known include lutein, lycopene, alpha-carotene, zeaxanthin and beta-carotene. Eat more spinach and leafy greens, for example – such as silver beet, kale or collards – and you tap into a rich supply of zeaxanthin and lutein to protect the eyes and probably the brain too from degeneration. In one study of 356 older people reported in the Journal of the American Medical Association, research found that eating good quantities of these leafy green vegetables – the equivalent of a large spinach salad each day – reduced the risk of macular degeneration by 43 percent. This is the age-related retinal disease that has you holding a menu at arm's length in order to read it.

The most highly studied carotenoid is beta-carotene. In fact, so enthusiastic were the scientists who first discovered the effects of beta-carotene about its ability to protect our health, that nutritional supplement companies were quick to jump on the bandwagon and produce supplements with high levels of beta-carotene – touting them as a virtual cure-all for just about everything. The problem is that these commercially minded chemists lost track of one of the most important principles of natural health and healing: synergy.

Beta-carotene, like the other phytochemicals, vitamins and minerals, exists in a very fine balance with other health-enhancing compounds found in nature. The moment you separate one chemical out and take it on its own without acknowledging this fact, you not only undermine some of its ability to enhance health, you may also create a situation of imbalance. This is why a few years after nutritionists oversold beta-carotene there were a number of health warnings about taking too much of it. In one study, for instance, beta-carotene supplementation on its own was shown to interfere with vitamin D absorption. In another, taking excessive amounts of beta-carotene indicated that this procedure can reduce the body's ability to absorb another very important carotenoid – lycopene. What matters most in nature as in human health is a balance. All of the carotenoids together with the vitamins, minerals and other plant factors for health, work best just the way nature provides them, in a splendid and highly complex balance, which we can neither fully understand nor replicate. The message is clear: build your daily meals around the colourful vegetable kingdom by eating salads, drinking juices, and cooking them in ways that preserve as much of their innate life-enhancing abilities as possible.

ASPARAGUS PREVENTS PROBLEMS

Asparagus has long been used in ayurvedic medicine as a remedy against indigestion. Not long ago researchers compared the therapeutic effect of asparagus with a commonly used drug in the prevention of nausea and hiatus hernia, heartburn and gastric acid reflux. They discovered that asparagus was just as effective as the common drug remedy, yet had no side effects.

Asparagus also has great diuretic properties. It stimulates the digestion and has long been used to alleviate rheumatism and arthritis. A member of the lily family, asparagus was used by the ancient Greeks to treat kidney and liver troubles. It is one of the best natural remedies for PMS-related bloating and a top source of folic acid, the antioxidant glutathione and vitamin C. All three are associated with reduced risk of cancer, age-related degenerative diseases and heart disease.

FENNEL

As well as containing potassium, fennel also contains phyto-oestrogens. These are the natural plant hormones that help protect us from the onslaught of the dangerous oestrogens in the environment and from the negative effects of oestrogen-based drugs, which are given far too often to women. As a result, fennel is a useful vegetable in helping not only to regulate menstruation but also to clear PMS. It even stimulates the flow of breast milk in nursing mothers. When you buy fennel, look for the fattest stems – they have more flavour and more phytohormones in them.

MAGIC MUSHROOMS

When it comes to the more exotic varieties of mushroom – those widely used in the Orient that are now beginning to be used in number in the West – you could hardly do better than make them a daily part of your meals. These include oyster mushrooms, enoki mushrooms and tree ears, as well as the immune-boosting medicinal mushrooms, shiitaki, maitake and reishi. These 'big three' have been used in Japan for over 4,000 years to nourish and cleanse the body, to tone it and bring a high level of energy. You may find it difficult to get hold of maitake and reishi mushrooms, but the rest are readily available either in oriental shops, health food shops or good supermarkets.

Among the many potent immune-building compounds that Asian mushrooms contain is one called lentinan, which strengthens the body against infection and degeneration. Studies have shown that lentinan is more effective than prescription drugs in fighting 'flu. It has even been shown to slow down the destructive effect of the Aids virus and the growth of cancer when fed to animals with tumours.

Eating oriental mushrooms is also good for your heart. Shiitakes contain more than one compound and reduce cholesterol levels. In one study of a group of women who were given a mere 75 g (3 oz) of shiitakes a day, their cholesterol levels were reduced by an average of 12 percent. As far as the reishi mushroom is concerned, this powerful fungus is able to do all these things, and more. Scientists find that it is rich in an anti-cancer compound called canthaxanthin – a particular carotenoid – as well as other substances including lanostan, which helps protect against allergies thanks to its ability to inhibit the release of histamines in the body.

ONIONS FOR IMMUNITY

Onions help prevent thrombosis and lower blood pressure that's too high. They also inhibit the growth of cancer cells – probably thanks to their high flavonoid content, including quercetin as well as coumarin and ellagic acid. Use them too whenever you can. They not only improve the flavour of the food you prepare, but eating them is a sure-fire way of protecting yourself from acute illness as well as bringing long-term strength and support to the immune system.

PEPPERED PAST

Peppers go back at least 7,000 years in their many forms: bell peppers, pimentos, cherry peppers, paprika, piquin, anaheim, jalapeno, chilli, cayenne and aji, to name a few. They became part of European fare when Columbus returned from their native New World and introduced them to the court. By the mid-sixteenth century they were being cultivated widely in Spain and Portugal. All peppers are rich in vitamins C and E and the carotenoids, helping protect against degeneration and the damaging effects of toxic chemicals in the environment. The hotter peppers are rich in the alkaloid capsaicin, which appears to decrease pain, enhance digestion and even detoxify the body, protecting it from 'flu and colds. Eat peppers raw as crudités, bake them and add them to soups and stews. Their magnificent colour and health-enhancing capacities are truly a wonder to behold.

A TOMATO A DAY

Two recent research projects – one carried out in Harvard University and the other at the Cancer Research Center in Hawaii – showed that men and women who eat large quantities of tomatoes are less than half as likely to die of cancer than those who don't. Second, in people who had cancer already, eating good quantities of tomatoes doubled participants' survival time. No one as yet knows exactly why this is, except that tomatoes are very rich in lycopene, one of the powerful, plant-based antioxidants, which improves mental as well as physical functioning and at the same time reduces the risk of degenerative diseases. Tomatoes also contain good quantities of glutathione, another potent antioxidant, which helps enhance immune functioning, slows down premature ageing and even helps prevent macular degeneration.

GRAINS AND SEEDS
GRAINS

For the past twenty years we have been urged to eat more and more grains. Science has known for a long time that diseases of nutritional deficiency such as beriberi and pellagra can be prevented by eating plenty of grains, which are themselves rich in B-complex vitamins, fibre, trace elements and – provided they are freshly milled – essential fatty acids. Grains also boast plant-based antioxidant compounds, which help protect the body's DNA from free-radical damage and therefore from degeneration and early ageing. Whole grains are rich in vitamin E, another important antioxidant and protector to the immune system. Finally, they contain a great deal of fibre to help ward off disease, control diabetes and fight obesity.

But there is another reason, too, why we have been so urged in recent decades to eat grains, and this is entirely an economic one. Convenience foods are based on large quantities of wheat and corn simply because these foods are enormously cheap and easy to manipulate in the manufacture of commercial products. As a result, anyone who has grown up in the last two or three generations and been fed on convenience foods is likely to have overloaded their system with certain grains – particularly wheat. Out of this a large number of people have developed wheat sensitivities (so-called food allergies). So true is this that I find that most people used to eating foods that are filled with flour and other products such as pasta, sauces, biscuits, breads and muffins, find that when they give up wheat-based products in favour of more fruits and vegetables their energies, most satisfyingly, soar.

The whole question of food allergy is a big one – far too wide in scope to deal with here. However, I've chosen not to put recipes that call for wheat flour or any kind of wheat (except wheat grass juice, which acts differently in the body) in this book. Not eating wheat dramatically improves the energy levels of most people. Look to some of the other less widely used grains such as rye, brown rice and wild rice, barley, oats and buckwheat (not really a grain at all, but rather an edible fruit seed from Asia).

Unless you are one of those string beans who doesn't seem to gain weight no matter what you eat, you're better off making grains a quarter (or even less) of your diet and emphasizing instead the fresh fruits and vegetables and good quality proteins. Making this change and making sure that many of the vegetables are eaten raw not only helps clear excess weight from the body without dieting, it heightens energy, relieves water retention and can improve many niggling problems – from minor aches and pains to skin problems.

SEED POWER

Nuts like almonds and seeds are high in fat. But the fat they contain helps decrease cholesterol levels and plays an important part in preventing cardiovascular disease. The two essential fatty acids prevalent in most nuts and seeds are linoleic acid and alpha linolenic acid. Linoleic acid is pretty easy to find in fresh foods: alpha linolenic is not so easy, since it is destroyed quickly in food processing. Fresh walnuts, linseeds and rapeseeds are full of it.

All of the essential fatty acids found in seeds and nuts – from almonds and sesames to sunflower seeds, pumpkin seeds, macadamias, pecans and walnuts – are important for the regulation of reproductive functions in the body as well. Get too little of them and your hair, nails and skin will suffer. If you have a tendency to allergies or menstrual disorders, insufficient essential fatty acids will make you highly prone to attacks.

There are other virtues to nuts and seeds too. Walnuts, for instance, have been shown to lower blood cholesterol levels and reduce blood lipids. Almonds significantly lower cholesterol in the blood. Macadamias, which are rich in a mono-unsaturated fatty acid, are linked to a reduction in high blood pressure and strokes in people who eat them in quantities. Brazils are rich in selenium too, so much so that a single Brazil nut offers enough of this vital antioxidant to meet the recommended daily allowance. This important mineral has been shown to enhance immunity and protect the body from free-radical damage. Nuts and seeds are also rich in isoflavones and in lignans. Recent studies show that pumpkin seeds may help reduce enlarged prostate glands because they are rich in specific amino acids that help clear symptoms of prostate trouble.

Pumpkin seeds are richer in zinc than any other plant – so important for good immunity, for growth, for wound healing and to make sure your sense of taste and smell works as it should. They are also a good source of iron, phosphorus, potassium and magnesium and they boast a huge amount of fibre – 10 g in each 25 g (1/4 oz in each 1 oz) of seeds – as well as some vitamin A. Sunflower seeds are a rich natural source of vitamin E and linoleic acid, both of which not only benefit the heart but help protect from premature ageing and degeneration. They have anti-cancer and anti-ageing potential thanks to their beta-carotene content and they support the adrenals, which helps enhance your ability to deal with stress. Eating only 30 g (just over 1 oz) of sunflower seeds a day will double most people's vitamin E intake.

Buy nuts and seeds raw, and preferably from stores that keep them refrigerated, since the essential fatty acids they contain are highly prone to rancidity. Once you get them home, make sure you keep them in the refrigerator. I find the best way to use nuts and seeds is to mix two or three types together. I often grind mine in a coffee grinder – since you can do a very small quantity at a time. You can keep ground nuts or seeds for a week or two at a time in tightly covered jars in the refrigerator.

SPROUT IT

As a seed sprouts, enzymes which have been dormant spring into action. The starches within the seeds are converted into natural sugars, proteins become amino acids and peptides and crude fats are broken down into fatty acids. In effect, the sprouting process pre-digests the food for you, turning these seeds into foods that are easily assimilated by your body when you eat them. Because of the massive enzyme release that occurs when a seed or grain is sprouted, the nutritional quality of a sprout is extremely good. These enzymes not only neutralize such factors as trypsin inhibitors but also destroy any other substances present that might be harmful.

Sprouts have many times the nutritional value of the seeds from which they have grown. They provide more nutrients gram for gram than any natural food known. During the sprouting process the vitamin content of seeds increases dramatically. For instance, the vitamin C content in soya beans multiplies five times within three days of germination. A mere tablespoon of soya bean sprouts contains half the recommended daily adult requirement of this vitamin. The vitamin B2 in an oat grain rises by 1,300 percent almost as soon as the seed germinates, and by the time tiny leaves have formed it has risen to 2,000 percent. Some sprouted seeds and grains are believed to have anti-cancer properties, which is why they form an important part in natural methods of treating the disease.

FIBRE MATTERS

Here is a list of different fibres, each of which works wonders for health in its own unique way:

Cellulose You find cellulose mostly in the outer layers of fruits and vegetables as well as in some nuts and grains. It has been shown to prevent constipation and haemorrhoids, and therefore varicose veins.

Gums and mucilages These kinds of fibre, which you find in seeds and grains, beans and many seaweeds, also lower blood cholesterol as well as help regulate glucose levels. They are particularly useful in clearing heavy metals, such as lead, from the body and removing other toxins.

Haemocellulose Found in vegetables, grains and fruits, a high level of haemocellulose in the diet has been shown to lower the risk of colon cancer by clearing many carcinogens from the intestines. It too is believed to help in weight loss.

Lignin Found in fruits and vegetables as well as in Brazil nuts, lignin helps prevent the formation of gallstones, lowers LDL cholesterol and reduces the risk of colon cancer. It can even help decrease the need for insulin in adult-onset diabetes.

Pectin This soluble fibre slows down the absorption of nutrients from meals. This means that it helps decrease appetite and is therefore useful for anyone wanting to shed excess fat. It also reduces the risk of heart disease, eliminates many toxins from the body – including dangerous heavy metals – and helps lower LDL cholesterol. You'll find pectin in citrus fruits and other fruits and vegetables as well as in dried peas.

NATURAL HELP

Herbs and sices are not totally flavoured-enhanceers - they can be fabulous health-enhancers too.

BASIL

Basil has some pretty remarkable healing properties. It calms the stomach and brings a soothing quality to the whole body. Basil is also rich in monoterpenes. These are phytonutrients with powerful antioxidant properties. It also has other plant chemicals, which soothe stomach cramps and calm upset stomachs, including eugenol – known for its ability to ease muscle spasms. Finally, basil is antiseptic and mildly sedative.

CHILLIES

Most people when they think of chillies think of herbs and spices not of health. But chillies are a great addition to a health-enhancing diet – even in the smallest doses. One chilli boasts 100 percent of the daily recommended dose of the antioxidant beta-carotene plus as much as 200 percent of that of vitamin C. Both these nutrients help fight free radicals and therefore help protect against heart disease, cancer and early ageing. They also strengthen immunity. In addition, chillies contain a plant chemical called capsaicin, which not only creates their fire but also helps prevent high LDL cholesterol in the blood.

Throughout history, chillies have been used to relieve pain as well. Recent research shows capsaicin has the ability to temporarily block chemically transmitted pain signals in the body. This is why you find it in natural ointments used to relieve arthritis and nerve pain. You will even find it in nose sprays helpful in clearing headaches. There is good evidence that capsaicin may even soothe pains of the mind and soul since it appears to trigger the release of the mood-enhancing endorphins in the brain.

FENUGREEK

Fenugreek is rich in diosgenin, a phytochemical from which chemists in the laboratory derive nature-identical progesterone. As a result, fenugreek is now also grown widely for the pharmaceutical industry. It enhances libido and helps clear premature ejaculation in men. Fenugreek also enhances digestion and is one of the best deep cleansers for the body that you can find in nature. It has a slightly spicy and bitter taste. When the leaves are very young and fresh they are a little bit like curry. I generally use the seeds to make tea.

GARLIC

Garlic has been prescribed for thousands of years as a cure for just about everything. But just in case this information has you running out for garlic pills, don't. It is much better to eat a couple of cloves of garlic a day in your food, either raw or lightly cooked. Garlic has much more powerful antibiotic properties when you eat it raw than when you cook it.

Here are some of its benefits.

 * Garlic lowers total cholesterol while increasing HDL (the 'good') cholesterol and reduces the susceptibility towards LDL (the so-called 'bad') cholesterol to oxidize. This oxidation process is the first step by which the arterial walls become damaged. One study showed that even 1/2 to 1 clove of garlic a day can lower cholesterol on average by 9 percent.

 * Lowers blood pressure. Garlic mimics the action of hypertensive drugs but has none of the side effects.

 * Blocks the ability of carcinogenic compounds to affect normal cells. This may be the means by which garlic inhibits the growth of cancer cells within the body.

 * Stimulates immune function. Garlic fights off many of the bacteria and fungi that medicine believes to be responsible for illness in humans. It also boosts the number of natural cure cells. Many epidemiological studies show a link between eating garlic frequently – as well as scallions, chives and onions – and a significant reduction in the risk of stomach cancer within a population.

 * Protects the cells against free-radical damage and therefore the body against premature ageing and degeneration.

 * Reduces the tendency of blood to clot and even helps dissolve existing clots once they've formed.

No wonder garlic has been prescribed for thousands of years as

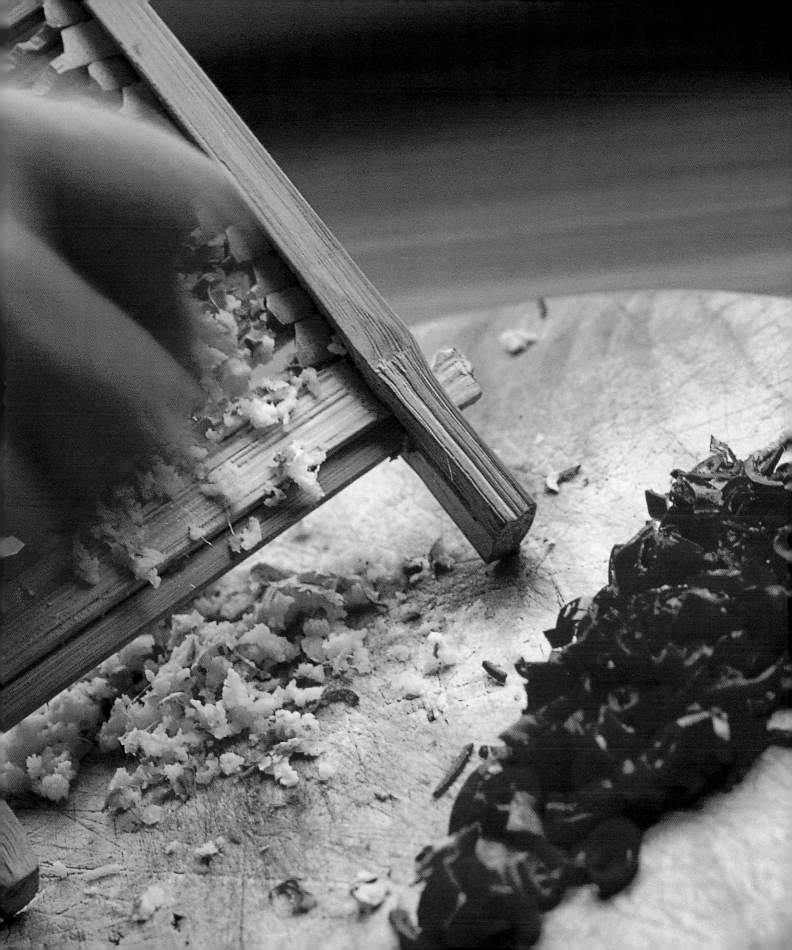

a cure for just about everything. But just in case this information has you running out for garlic pills, don't. It is much better to eat a couple of cloves of garlic a day in your food, either raw or lightly cooked. Garlic has much more powerful antibiotic properties when you eat it raw than when you cook it.

GLORIOUS GINGER

The spicy sweet ginger root is one of the greatest of all the natural health enhancers of the vegetable kingdom. It is not only well known for its ability to calm an upset stomach and banish travel sickness — better, in fact, than the well-known over-the-counter medicine Dramamine. Ginger is also brilliant at alleviating the symptoms of colds and flu; it increases circulation, and calms fevers. It even helps PMS and headaches and has heart-protecting properties thanks to its ability to discourage the clumping of blood cells.

To help prevent nausea all you need to take is half a teaspoon of dried ginger or a tiny piece of fresh ginger. It relieves indigestion and flatulence. Ginger stimulates circulation and is used in natural medicine to counter rheumatism. In a study done in Denmark in 1992 researchers confirmed what ayurvedic practitioners have long insisted, that ginger relieves the pain of arthritis and rheumatism without side effects. Many scientists studying this amazing root believe that ginger works its wonders thanks to an ability to block inflammatory tendencies in the body.

ROSEMARY REVIVES

Rosemary has a natural ability to soften the skin. When used in a carrier and rubbed on the body its essential oils are a great help in relieving muscular soreness. But what I like best about rosemary is the way it revitalizes the senses.

GO FISH

Part of the reason why fish is so wonderful is that it is rich in polyunsaturated omega-3 fatty acids. A high level of these essential fatty acids in the diet is associated with very low levels of stroke as well as a decreased risk of every sort of heart disease. In part, this is because these EFAs make the blood less likely to clot. They also help lower blood pressure, reduce triglycerides — the fats that circulate in the blood — and decrease the levels of the low-density lipoproteins (BLDL) and cholesterol, which in turn reduces the tendency that blood platelets have to clump and build up on the artery walls. Omega-3 fatty acids also inhibit the progress of breast cancer and help prevent tumours in general. The best sources of omega-3 fatty acids are cold-water fish such as anchovies, sardines, swordfish, bass, mackerel and wild salmon. Even

oysters and squid are high in omega-3.

In the average diet, the ratio of omega-3 to omega-6 fatty acids tends to be about 1:10, a ratio which most nutritional experts believe is highly dangerous to health. When the level of omega-6 is higher in the body than omega-3, this triggers an increase in some prostaglandins and leucotrines — substances like hormones that decrease immune function, encourage the formation of blood clots and can produce heart rhythms that are irregular. Much better for health is a balance of 50:50 omega-3 and omega-6 fatty acids.

I use a product called Udo's Choice, which is a beautiful balance of omega-3 and omega-6 fatty acids (see Resources). In Udo's Choice, the omega-3s are not taken from fish, but rather from cold-pressed vegetable oils. It was developed by the Canadian expert in essential fatty acids Udo Erasmus. And although there are many copies on the market, Udo's Choice is still the best worldwide both for purity and for taste. You can buy it in the best health food stores. It must be kept chilled in the refrigerator at all times, and you need to use it within a few weeks, as all the essential fatty acids are highly prone to degeneration. One thing more: never heat it. Use it for salad dressings, pour it over cooked potatoes or vegetables. Mix it with soft butter then chill and spread it on bread instead.

There is more to the fish oil story too. Two compounds in fish oil, eicosapentaenoic acid (EPA) and docosahexaenoic acid (DHA), both of which are rich in fish oils, are known to help prevent the build-up of plaque on the walls of the arteries. They even help mitigate the destructive effects of a diet high in fat. Surprisingly enough, both EPA and DHA have also been shown to relieve pain in people with rheumatoid arthritis and decrease the number of headaches in migraine sufferers.

GO FOR ANCHOVIES

Anchovies are a great source of omega-3 fatty acids. These fatty acids, which are virtually impossible to come by on a diet of convenience foods, have been shown to inhibit the growth of cancer tumours and may also help lower soaring blood cholesterol levels. Anchovies are also rich in the nucleic acids DNA and RNA, which some experts in human biochemistry believe may help prevent premature ageing. They appear to help the body create healthy and long-lived cells.

MUSSELS HAVE MUSCLE

With their beautiful blue-green shells, these sea gems, when harvested from unpolluted waters, are not only a highly nutritious form of protein, they are rich in vitamins and trace minerals as well as an excellent source of mucopolysaccharides and the free-radical scavenging enzyme superoxide dismutase. Extracts of the green-lipped mussel have been used successfully to treat inflammatory diseases from rheumatoid and osteoarthritis to eczema and emphysema. Recently they have even taken their place in the growing arsenal of natural cancer treatments.

PRAWNS FOR SKIN

The shells are filled with chitin – a protein substance that cosmetic manufacturers now use to strengthen skin from both within and without. Like most shellfish, prawns are rich in iodine and in the antioxidants zinc and selenium.

Prawns are excellent for people who eat very little, thanks to their being an easily digested form of top quality protein. They are also a good source of calcium and the important omega-3 fatty acids, which offer not only protection for the heart but good support for hormonal health and skin health and beauty too.

SEXY OYSTERS

Oysters as an aphrodisiac got much of their good press from Casanova, who consumed an average of 40 of these sea gems each day. And there is a scientific basis for Casanova's claims. Not only are oysters a good source of protein – very important for the production of reproductive hormones – they are also a rich source of iodine, which is necessary for the proper functioning of the thyroid gland. If the thyroid is deficient, libido lessens and then gently fades away. The thyroid in many ways keeps the other glands in the body working as they should do. Oysters are also an excellent source of vitamin B12, vitamin E and niacin, as well as potassium, iron and selenium. They are also the richest natural source of zinc. In fact, just six raw oysters provide over five times the recommended daily amount of zinc. This is important because zinc is essential for the production of sperm. Also, zinc is believed to enhance libido. Finally, recent research into foods from the sea indicates that certain sterols are present in oysters as well as other molluscs, from which both the sex hormones and cortisone are derived.

When buying oysters, make sure you get them from a reliable source. Scrub their shells well in clean water and try to eat them the day that you purchase them. Always make sure that the shells are closed. Tap any open oyster shells with a knife and if they don't close, discard them. In many countries in the Northern Hemisphere it has long been illegal to harvest native oysters in the summer when they are spawning. Nowadays, however, Pacific oysters are commercially farmed in Britain so that you can enjoy oysters all year round.

CLEANSING SEAWEEDS

All seaweeds are marine algae – the oldest form of life on the planet; and most of them have something in common. They are filled with soothing mucilaginous gels such as algin, agar and carrageen. They alkalinize the blood. They help clear liver stagnation and therefore, from the point of view of oriental medicine, help activate the chi – the body's life energy – when we eat them. Seaweeds are excellent lymphatic cleansers. Even in small quantities they supply biologically available minerals and trace elements as nothing else can. From 5 to 15 g (1/8 to 1/2 oz) of sea plants a day (measured before soaking or cooking) will supply you with a broad range of minerals – so broad that it's unlikely that, unless you have a specific high requirement for particular minerals, you will need to take any mineral supplements. Kelp, kombu and arami seaweeds contain from 100 to 500 times more iodine than does shellfish, and up to 3,000 times the iodine of fish itself – vital for the health of the thyroid and for optimum metabolic functioning. Arame, wakame and hijiki seaweeds boast more than ten times the calcium of milk. Kelp and wakame contain more than four times the iron found in the best beef steak.

It is the orientals who have made the best use of seaweeds in their foods. However, in peasant traditions in Europe and the United States, you also find many seaweeds. Bladder wrack, for instance, sea lettuce and kelp make good soups. The only problem with seaweeds – and it's a big one – is that you need to make sure the sea plants you eat come from seas that are relatively unpolluted, particularly by heavy metals, since wherever seaweeds grow they tend to accumulate whatever metals and minerals are in the waters. When you first introduce seaweeds to your diet it's a good idea to do it slowly, as it sometimes takes a week or two for the body to get used to digesting sea vegetables. Their flavour is also unique. For a few people it takes a bit of getting used to.

SEA GELATINE

The sea vegetable derivative, agar agar, is made out of the mucilaginous fibre from several seaweeds, many of which grow to great size. In the Orient it is used to promote weight loss and to improve digestion. It's a great source of both iron and calcium, and it makes wonderful fruit gels. However you take them, if you've never used sea vegetables for cooking, this is an ideal time to begin. A whole new world of flavour and texture awaits exploration. The Japanese call it kanten, and it has a particular ability to gel. The seaweeds from which agar agar is made are known collectively as agarophytes, the most important of which is a seaweed called gelidium, which grows as deep as 60 m (200 ft), waving its huge leaves in the sea. Perhaps a thousand years ago the Japanese discovered how to dehydrate the fronds so that they became transparent and could be made into kanten bars that one could use as easily as gelatine.

In many ways, agar agar is far superior to gelatine. However, it has a much firmer texture and it does not easily melt. It is also calorie free and for vegetarians is ideal, as it is a completely natural vegetable product. Not only that, but this wonderful gift from the sea has a slightly sweet flavour and benefits the body in many ways — by reducing inflammation, strengthening the heart and lungs and through its mildly laxative action. The Japanese use it to encourage weight loss and even to carry toxic and radioactive waste out of the body. Finally, it is an excellent dietary source of both calcium and iron.

EGGS MATTER
Eggs are a great food — a superb source of top quality protein among other things. It is a pity that for so long they were wrongly accused of raising cholesterol levels. The protein they offer is just about the best you can get apart, maybe, from fresh raw fish or raw organic liver. (And not many people are drawn to eating raw organic liver.) Rich in the sulphur-based amino acids, eggs have excellent antioxidant properties to help protect you from free-radical damage that leads to degeneration and early ageing as well. Such sulphur amino acids need to be available for the body to make its own natural free-radical-fighting enzymes such as glutathione peroxidase. Eggs are also full of antioxidant vitamins A and E as well as vitamins D and B12 and lecithin. An emulsifier essential to good brain functioning, lecithin has been shown to enhance memory, mood and concentration. Finally, eggs are truly satisfying. They 'stick to your ribs'. Their protein-based energy is released slowly into the bloodstream. This makes them great for breakfast. They help guard against blood sugar ups and downs that have you reaching for another cup of coffee or a sticky bun at 11am.

SOYA GUARDS
Populations who regularly consume soya products have reduced rates of breast cancer, colon cancer and prostate cancer. Why? The soya bean is rich in phyto-hormones — plant-based oestrogens such as the isoflavones genistein and daedzein. Unlike the dangerous xenoestrogen chemicals from petrochemically derived herbicides, pesticides and plastics in our environment — which lower male sperm count and wreak havoc with women's reproductive systems — soya's plant hormones are gentle.

When we eat foods rich in phyto-oestrogens, like soya, these weak plant hormones are taken up by the oestrogen receptor sites in our body, where they help protect us from the uptake of dangerous cancer-inducing xenoestrogens all around us. In effect, if you eat a good quantity of the phyto-oestrogens you go a long way towards protecting yourself from the reproductive damage and the higher susceptibility to cancer and degeneration that has resulted in recent years from rising environmental pollution.

There are many other health claims now being made for soya products as well. Most of them are proving to be true. The isoflavin daedzein, for example, is a metabolite, which helps prevent the decrease in bone mass that leads to osteoporosis. Along with the isoflavones, soya is rich in saponins and other phytosterols, which help lower cholesterol levels, either by blocking cholesterol absorption or by enhancing your body's ability to get rid of any excess. This is probably why soya is often credited with an ability to reduce the risk of cardiovascular disease in people who eat it frequently.

Long-term consumption of a mere 30 to 50 mg a day of isoflavones has been shown to lower the risk of heart disease. As in the case of other health-enhancing phytochemicals such as the carotenoids, flavonoids and antioxidants, there is a powerful synergistic effect in getting the protective isoflavones, saponins and other plant chemicals all together as nature packaged them in soya beans. They work synergistically. When it comes to the good effects they bring, the whole is greater than the sum of the parts. There is simply no way to create in a nutritional supplement the fine synergy that natural soya bean foods offer. Just one serving of soya a day is a great strategy for lowering your risk of degenerative diseases and protecting yourself from the carcinogenic effects of environmental chemicals. A serving of soya only consists of 250 ml (8 fl oz) of soya milk or 50 g (2 oz) of soya beans, tofu or tempeh.

One word of warning, however. Soya beans, like corn and tomato products, have been highly genetically engineered in recent years and there is a powerful argument against eating any genetically engineered products. We have no idea what the long-term effects of eating products that have been artificially manipulated will be. But in most countries, provided you choose organic foods, you should be safe from any genetically engineered products — another good reason to eat organic.

MEET GOOD MEAT
All forms of meat contain high levels of protein and an abundance of minerals and trace minerals. Wild game is low in

fat – much lower than pork, lamb or beef – and the fat itself is highly unsaturated, very much like fish fat. Partridge, venison, grouse and quail are all higher in iron than any other meat except for offal, such as liver and heart. They are also extremely rich in zinc as well as vitamins B6, B12 and B2, niacin and pantothentic acid.

The problem with domestic meats is that in many countries most of them are laden with hormones, toxins and antibiotics. When you routinely eat large quantities of meat you can end up not only with a high level of uric acid in your body, but also with a tendency to form a lot of mucus and to build up toxicity. This is why, when I eat meat – and I prefer fish or game – I eat certified organic meat. The difference in flavour is remarkable and I know that the animals that I'm eating have been carefully raised and are free of both excess fat and the toxicity that most domestic farm animals carry these days.

I was a vegetarian for twenty years and I still believe that a vegetarian diet is ideal for many people. I discovered, however, in my mid-thirties that vegetarianism was not ideal for me – probably because my ancestors, being Nordic, spent most of their lives living on fish, salted meat and whatever cabbage they could dig up from the frozen ground. Our genetic make-up determines to a great extent what works for us and what doesn't. When I added fish and game to my meals, my energy levels soared and I looked and felt better.

Each of us is unique. This not only determines what kind of foods we thrive on, it also determines what kinds of foods are best for us at any particular time of our life. Many women at menopause, for instance, find they do much better by cutting meat out of their diet. Others discover just the opposite – that they need more protein. It's a question of 'suck it and see'. Don't hesitate to shift from eating more fruit at one time of your life to more vegetables at another, and more fish at another. The human body is always changing, as are our needs for various foods.

COFFEE PROS AND CONS

Despite the warnings in recent years about how dangerous coffee is to health – and there is truth in many of them – coffee also has benefits to mind and body. For instance, it has been prescribed for generations in the treatment of asthma, vertigo, headaches, jaundice and even snake bite. A poultice of wet coffee grounds speeds the healing of insect stings and bruises. Coffee enemas are used as a strong purgative stimulant both to the bowels and to the liver in the natural treatment of serious illness, including cancer.

Coffee is here to stay. The challenge then becomes how we make the most of what it offers while ensuring that our health is not undermined by drinking it. Let's look at the dangers first.

Research shows that women who drink coffee while eating a high-fat diet, have a greater risk of both breast cancer and bladder cancer. Similarly, drinking coffee during pregnancy increases the rate of birth defects and miscarriages. Even moderate coffee drinking can raise cholesterol levels in some people. From the point of view of digestion, coffee has a tendency to eat away the villi in the small intestine. This, in turn, can interfere with assimilation of nutrients from food – one of the reasons why heavy coffee drinkers tend to be deficient in minerals including calcium. Another reason lies in coffee's acidity. When the body becomes too acidic from drinking a lot of coffee, it tends to leach calcium – an alkaline element – from the bones to balance the acidity of the blood.

Virtually all of the research into the damaging effects of coffee has been done using readily available coffee in the market-place, almost all of which is contaminated by an ever-increasing number of herbicides and pesticides. These can build up to poison the body by interfering with metabolic processes. In so-called developed countries, such as Europe and the United States, once a herbicide or pesticide is labelled 'dangerous to human health' it is made illegal. But the chemical companies who produce it then tend to send the banned chemical to Third World countries for use there. Coffee, of course, is grown in Third World countries – in most of which there are no statutory controls over how much of a specific herbicide or pesticide can be sprayed on crops. As a result, coffee is one of the most contaminated foods in the world.

I take with a grain of salt some of the negative results of the scientific research that's been done into how damaging coffee is to the human body. I strongly suspect that much of the damage may be due not to the caffeine, as is commonly supposed, but to the chemical contamination that the coffee beans carry. This makes the argument for organic coffee a strong one. Coffee grown organically tends to be grown in a way that, unlike conventionally grown, does not exploit the native peoples who work in the coffee plantations, but rather gives them fair financial remuneration for their work. Also, organic coffee is free of the chemical dangers, none of which have been fully investigated but which are certainly considerable in relation to human health. So, when buying coffee, go organic, it also has a finer flavour than the coffees that are grown with herbicides and pesticides.

LOVE IN THE AFTERNOON

6

The sun's chains hidden all among the leaves. Slivers of light through half-closed blinds. A glass of champagne and love. What part can food play in all this? A big one provided the foods are as primordial as love itself. Strawberries dipped in honey; oysters on the half shell; caviar with black bread and a slice of lemon, a simple glass of raspberry and ginseng tea. Many foods affect hormones, libido, energy and joy. Food for love is not so much a meal as an interlude with one or two vibrant foods or drinks, be they double chocolate brownies or something as simple as a splendid fruit salad spiked with the psychoactive nutmeg.

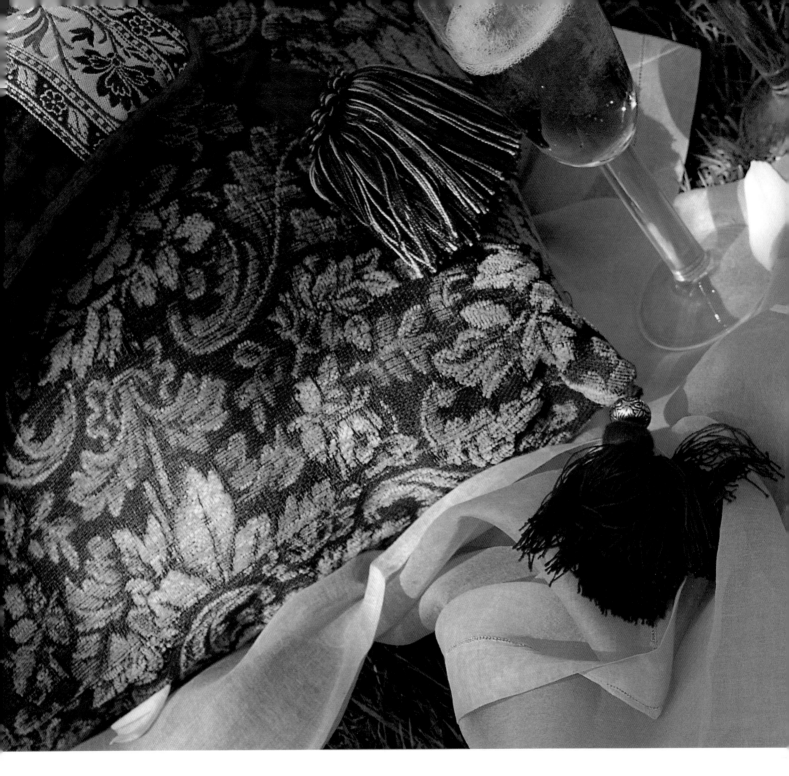

IF FOOD BE THE MUSIC OF LOVE, # EAT ON ...

OYSTERS ON THE HALF SHELL WITH CHABLIS

My favourite foods are caviar and popcorn with oysters and wild ruccola (or rocket) trailing close behind. Why? Who knows. The sensuousness of oysters, their wonderful colour and unique texture never ceases to delight me. The best in the world come from South Africa. They are smaller than European oysters but so sweet that the first taste is always surprising. Always buy oysters alive. When dead, they deteriorate rapidly and can be dangerous. Know their origin. Make sure they come from clean water. A live oyster will be tightly shut. If one is slightly open, touch it. If it doesn't close immediately, throw it away. Once you have bought them, keep the oysters cold. This slows down their metabolism. A good oyster should feel heavy and sound full if you tap its shell. To get the very best from them, eat them as soon as they are well chilled. (For the Inside Story on oysters, see page 93.)

SIMPLY OYSTERS

serves 2

WHAT YOU NEED
2 dozen fresh oysters, checked and scrubbed
a good oyster knife
1 bottle of ice-cold Chablis
a few wedges of lemon

HERE'S HOW
With an oyster knife open each oyster, being careful not to lose the juice from the inside. Lay on a plate or even a bed of crushed ice if you happen to have it. Serve immediately on a large platter with lemons and sauce on the side. Two white damask napkins come in handy here too, since eating oysters can be a liquid affair.

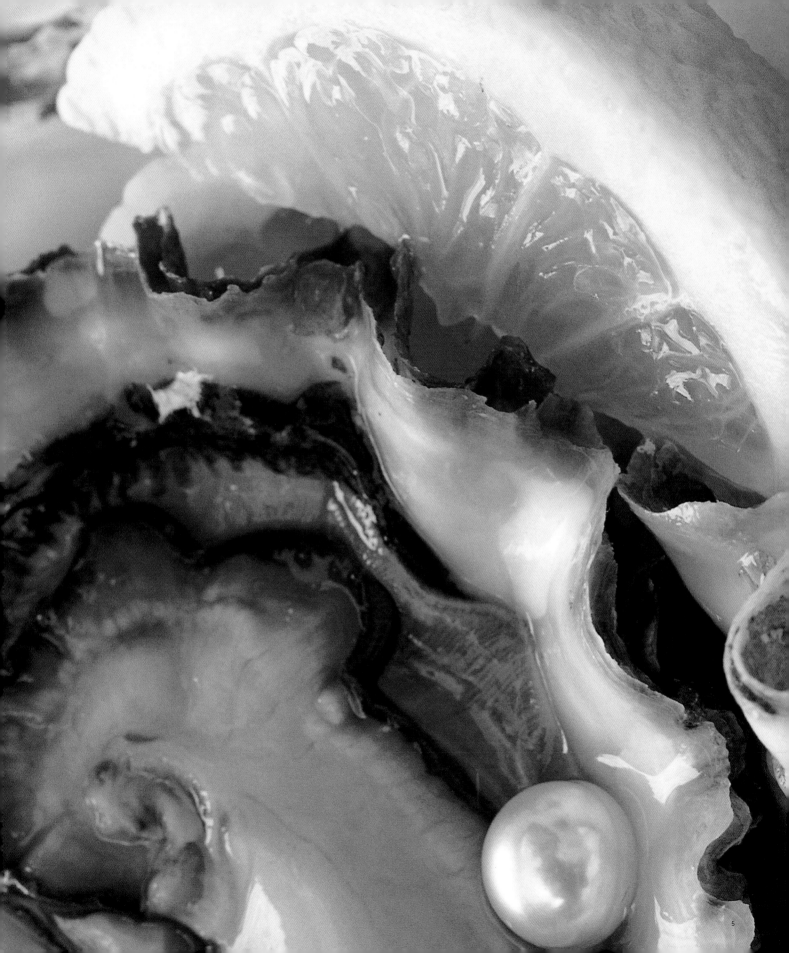

5

ZHOUG SAUCE FOR OYSTERS

This sauce, which comes from the Yemen, adds a real bite to the oyster. You make it as hot or as mild as you wish.

WHAT YOU NEED

120 g (4 1/2 oz) fresh coriander
1-3 medium-hot chillies, de-
    seeded and finely chopped
seeds of 8 cardamom pods,
    crushed
5 tbsp extra-virgin olive oil
Maldon sea salt and freshly
    ground pepper
6 garlic cloves, finely chopped
zest of 1/2 lemon, finely
    shredded

HERE'S HOW

Add all of the ingredients, except the finely chopped garlic, zest of lemon and one quarter of finely chopped fresh coriander, to a food processor. Blend well, then pour into a dish and add the chopped garlic, lemon zest and the remaining coriander. Chill well and serve in a small dish with a spoon so that you can spoon the sauce over the oysters as you wish.

CAVIAR IN BED

The wonderful things about caviar are the way it pops in the mouth as you eat it and the way each kind has a completely different flavour. Red, black, silver … I love them all. I used to have a friend who often travelled to Russia and the Middle East. He would return from trips with his suitcases stuffed with ripe mangoes and caviar by the kilo bought on the black market – from pilots who fly the route often and become tired of the stuff. (This is something I simply can't imagine.) I love caviar served with thinly sliced 100 percent German rye bread maybe spread with sweet butter. But I love it too served with organic raw carrot sticks, celery and fresh fennel. I even adore it on fresh apple slices. I often serve it with a little bowl of chopped onions and another of chopped hard-boiled eggs. Just dip and eat.

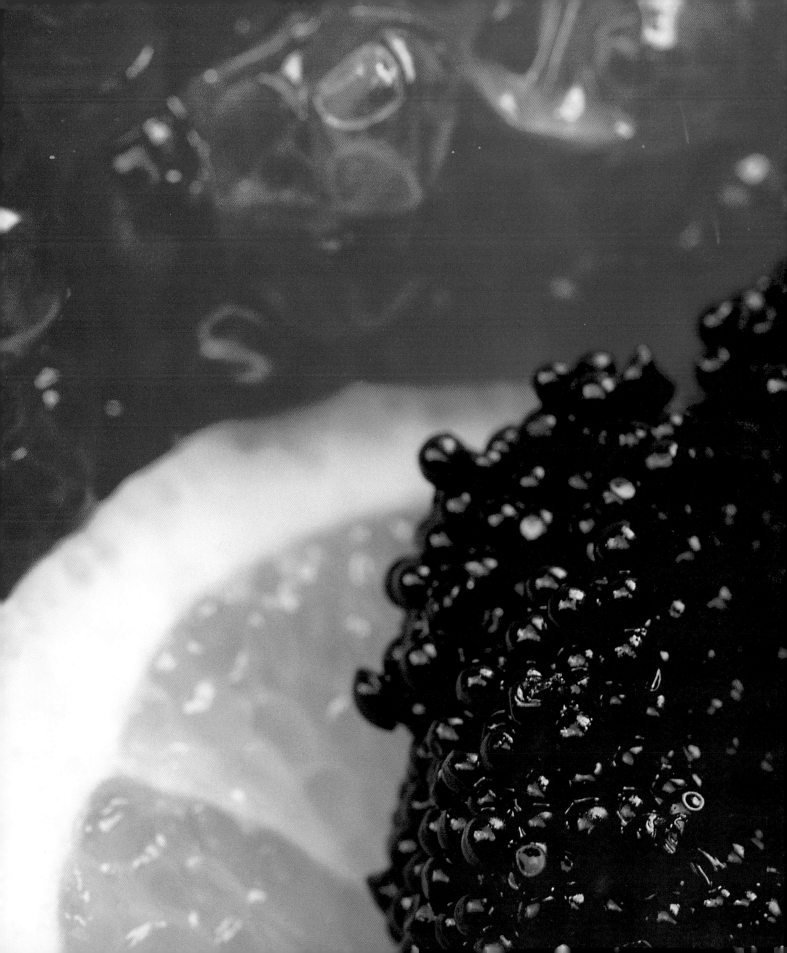

SEX AND ALCOHOL

There is no question that alcohol in small doses stimulates desire. In excess, it's a real sexual downer - especially for men. The question becomes just how much alcohol is ideal and what kind is best? In medicine, the desirable dose of any active ingredient in a drug depends upon the ratio between its helpful effect and the point at which it becomes toxic to the body. This is known as the therapeutic to toxic ratio. So it is with alcohol.

The champagne experience

One of the best alcoholic drinks in the world for intensifying sexual pleasure is champagne. Champagne bottles are corked after the first fermentation. This causes the second fermentation to produce a great deal of carbon dioxide, which, as it builds up, creates this sparkling wine. It also creates other compounds including tyramine. Tyramine is a plant substance, found in mature cheeses, red wine, chocolate and fava beans as well as in champagne, which has a stimulating effect. It is something that a few people, especially those who suffer from migraine and food intolerance or are on anti-depressant drugs, need to avoid, since it in turn causes the release of histamine from mast cells in the body and can create allergic reactions.

But the positive side of tyramine is that it brings about the release of catecholamines in the body. These are uplifting stimulating compounds that belong to a larger family of substances including the hormones adrenalin and noradrenalin a well as dopamine, which excite the peripheral muscles and intensify the beating of the heart as well as affecting other metabolic functions involved in making love. These hormones also stimulate the action of the endocrine glands and, in a healthy person, bring a feeling of uplift to the whole nervous system. It may be this stimulation leading both to physical excitation and also to a talkativeness that is so much a part of the champagne experience, which makes it such a good thing for love - and why it has long had the reputation as a truth serum.

CHAMPAGNE AND KIWI FRUIT GRANITA

serves 2

This granita gets its colour from the fruit itself. It's important when you make this granita that you use ripe kiwi fruit. The texture of the fruit with its dark seeds makes an unusually beautiful and uplifting dessert.

What you need

250 ml (8 fl oz) fresh kiwi fruit pulp

450 ml (16 fl oz) good champagne

1 tbsp lime zest, finely shredded

2-3 tsp honey or golden granulated sugar

fresh mint to garnish (optional)

HERE'S HOW

Peel, then purée the kiwi fruit, making sure you get 250 ml (8 fl oz) of purée. Combine the pulp with the other ingredients, blending well. To make the granita in a freezer, place the mixture in a freezer tray and freeze until solid. Remove and break into large chunks with a fork. Finally purée the chunks in a food processor until they go smooth and creamy. Return to the freezer for another 30 minutes. Serve by itself in simple bowls.

SENSUOUS FRUIT

Fruit is sexy. Don't let anybody tell you otherwise. And bed is a favourite place to eat it with a lover - even with a special friend. Dip gigantic strawberries into pale gold acacia honey. Share a juicy mango. Half the fun of it is the game of trying to keep yourself - and the sheets - dry as you do.

BERRIES PURE AND SIMPLE

serves 2

Try fresh blueberries and raspberries smothered in a simple sauce of whipped raspberries and maple syrup eaten from one dish with your fingers.

ROSE PETAL AND GINGER COULIS

makes 250 ml (8 fl oz)

This beautiful sauce depends upon using the right kind of roses – the best flowers are either the deep red miniature varieties or large white heavily scented petals from old-fashioned roses. It is important to let the colour of the sauce develop in the refrigerator for four or five days if you are using apple juice. If you choose berries instead, the colour is already present and you can serve it right away. If you can't get the miniature red roses for this, you can use larger roses, but in that case you want to cut them into small pieces. You can drizzle this sauce, hot or cold, on ice cream or fresh fruit.

WHAT YOU NEED

handful rose petals plus a
  handful more picked just
  before serving as a garnish
2.5 cm (1 in) piece of fresh
  ginger, finely grated
1/2 tsp lemon juice
4 tbsp Muscat wine
175 g (6 oz) golden granulated
  sugar
125 ml (4 fl oz) crushed
  berries or apple juice
10 drops rosewater

HERE'S HOW

Mix all the ingredients, except the rosewater, and bring them to the boil. Simmer gently for 3 or 4 minutes. Now cool and add the rosewater. If you are using apple juice, store in the refrigerator for five days so the colour develops. Serve over mixed berries or other fruit, custard, or even chocolate brownies littered with more rose petals.

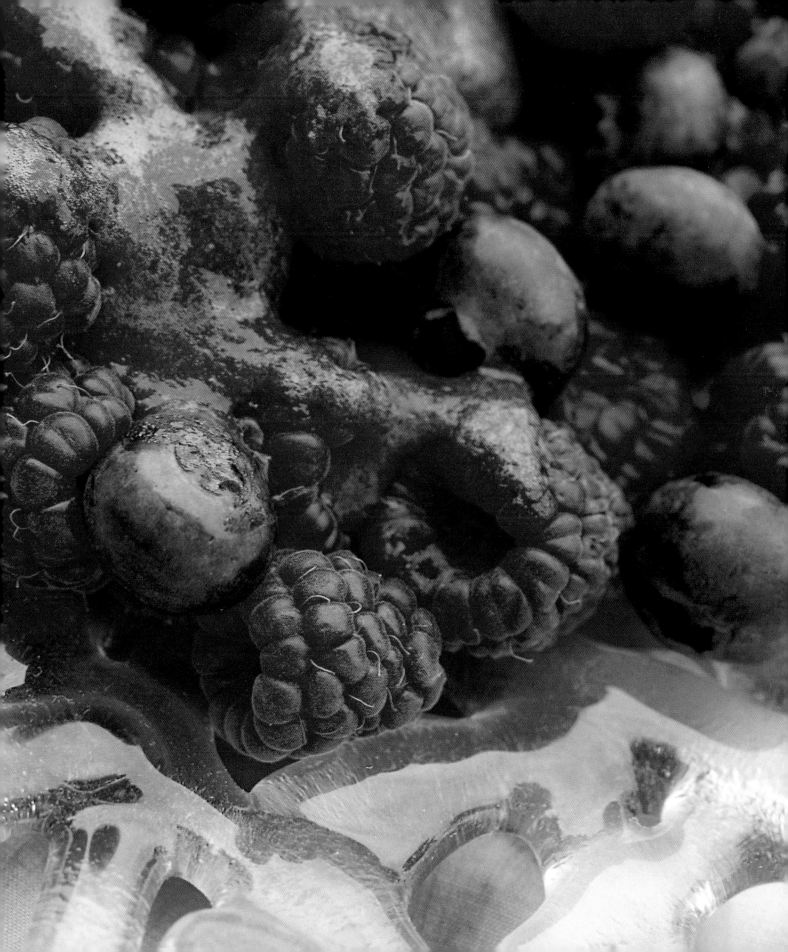

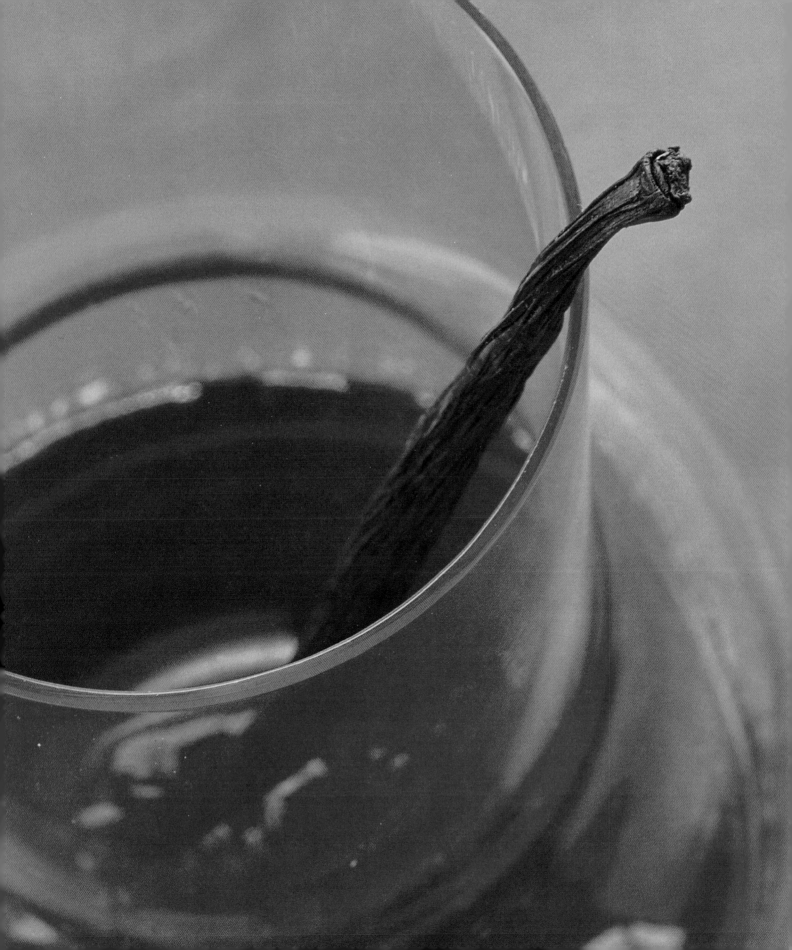

RASPBERRY, GINSENG AND VANILLA TEA

serves 2

Ginseng is full of phytosteroids - natural plant chemicals that not only improve our ability to deal with stress, but also act as mild sexual stimulants. Vanilla beans contain vanillin - also a mild stimulant. Raspberries are rich in potassium and not only beautiful to look at but soothing to the spirit. A combination of the three is hard to beat. You can serve this tea either hot or cold. The colour is like a summer sunset and the taste is sensuous beyond belief.

WHAT YOU NEED
100 g (4 oz) raspberries, either fresh or frozen
300 ml (10 fl oz) boiling water
1/2 tsp dried ginseng root, crushed, or a bag of good ginseng tea or a packet of freeze-dried ginseng granules
2 vanilla beans
4 tbsp maple syrup or acacia honey

HERE'S HOW
Wash the fruit. Put the raspberries in a saucepan with enough water to cover the base of the pan to prevent burning. Simmer over a low heat to extract the flavour from the raspberries. Strain into a cup and put aside. Put the ginseng and the vanilla in a teapot and pour boiling water over them. Steep for 3 minutes.

Add the maple syrup or honey and the raspberry mixture, strain. Rinse the vanilla bean and place in a tall tea glass or cup. Fill each cup with the mixture and serve immediately. You can also chill this and keep it in the refrigerator. I generally add a few more raspberries and a little more ginseng if I chill it, because things tend to lose their flavour when they are iced. If chilled, serve it over crushed ice.

WHITE MAGIC PESTO WITH BLACK BREAD

makes 450 g (1 lb)

Fava beans - otherwise known as broad beans, butter beans or white beans - are said to have whipped the Roman poet Cicero into a passion. Women have long known their secret: they are an awesome aphrodisiac. Science has just discovered why. White beans are probably the best food source of L-dopa, a neurotransmitter that uplifts the spirits and, among other things, encourages a firm erection.

Make use of the magical properties of butter beans by mixing them with the sensuous aroma of fresh basil - another renowned aphrodisiac. The recipe uses caramelized garlic to give it an earthy flavour. Serve warm or cold with fresh vegetables to scoop up generous mouthfuls. It is almost too sexy.

I use fresh broad beans or dried beans and soak them overnight. You can make this pesto in advance - even a day or two ahead - if you are that well organized. Put a little olive oil on the top to seal it and keep in an airtight container in the refrigerator. I use a lot of garlic cloves in this recipe, but you might prefer to start with fewer.

WHAT YOU NEED

175 g (6 oz) fresh broad beans
   or dried white beans, or a
   small can butter beans
6 garlic cloves
200 g (7 oz) fresh basil
   leaves
2 tbsp lemon juice
1-2 tbsp extra-virgin olive oil
1-2 tbsp powdered bouillon
Maldon sea salt and freshly
   ground pepper

HERE'S HOW

If you are using dried beans, soak them overnight in plenty of water. Rinse the soaked beans, put them in a pan and cover with 5 cm (2 in) of water. Cook gently for an hour or until tender, making sure there is always enough water to cover them. Let them cool. At the same time cook the garlic. Rub a tiny amount of olive oil on to a baking tray and lay out the peeled cloves of garlic. Bake them in the oven for about 40 minutes, turning them over occasionally, until

they are golden brown and soft. Allow
to cool.

Put the garlic, beans, basil,
lemon juice, 1 tablespoon of oil and
1 to 2 tablespoons of broth in a food
processor and blend until smooth. If
it is too thick, add a little more
oil and broth until you have a good
consistency. Season with salt and
black pepper, and serve with thick
slices of whole grain European rye
bread or with crudités.

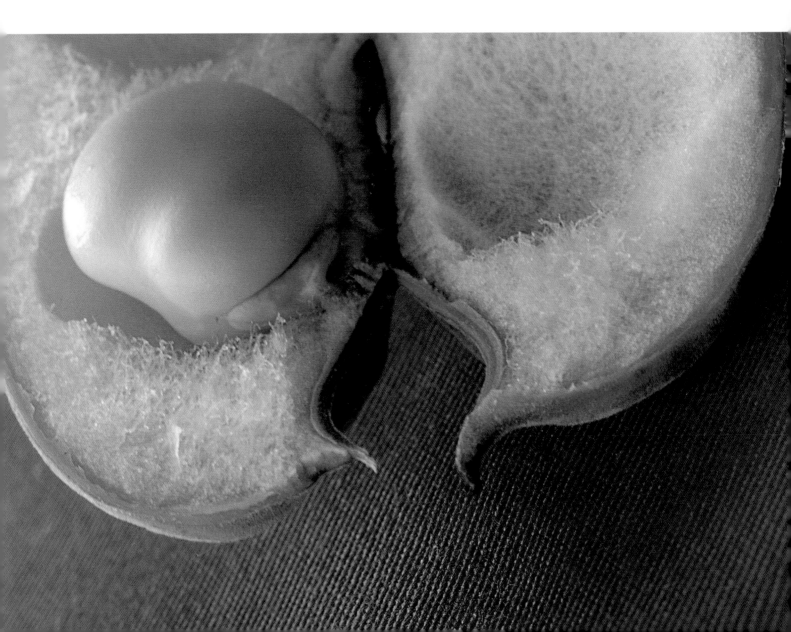

PSYCHO-SEXUAL CHOCOLATE

The mythology of chocolate began with the ancient gods of the New World. It was the Olmec Indians in Central America who are credited with the discovery of the cocoa tree. Later the Aztecs and Toltecs, who called this substance food of the gods, told the story of how Quetzalcoatl, the supreme God of the Air, brought the seeds of the tree to earth **as a gift to his chosen people. Montezuma the great Aztec king is believed to have downed 50 pitchers of an elixir made from chocolate each day. The drink was called xocolatl,** an aphrodisiac and fountain of strength, sexuality and vigour.

Only the best is good enough

Cortez, who brought it back to Europe in the sixteenth century, soon created a chocolate storm among the courtiers. Madame de Pompadour gave her seal of approval to chocolate as an aphrodisiac while Casanova claimed chocolate was the perfect tool for seduction. Some recent research partly explains why. Scientists in California have isolated a substance in chocolate that links into our brain receptor sites and, like cannabis, brings sensations of pleasure and relaxation. But chocolate, I suspect, has many secrets. And this is just one of them, which feeds our passion for this dark and seductive food and at the same time enhances our passion for love.

If you're going to eat chocolate, eat only the best, not only because it's the most delicious, but also because it is the real thing. On the market these days you find all sorts of imitation chocolate products, which have had vegetable fat added to them. Avoid them. Even natural chocolate is often processed with an alkali that makes it high in sodium and interferes with the absorption of the magnesium, copper, potassium, phosphorus, iron and calcium which are the natural birthright of pure cocoa. When buying chocolate, always buy plain chocolate or bitter, dark chocolate, and always go organic. There is no question whatsoever that organic chocolate is the most delicious in the world.

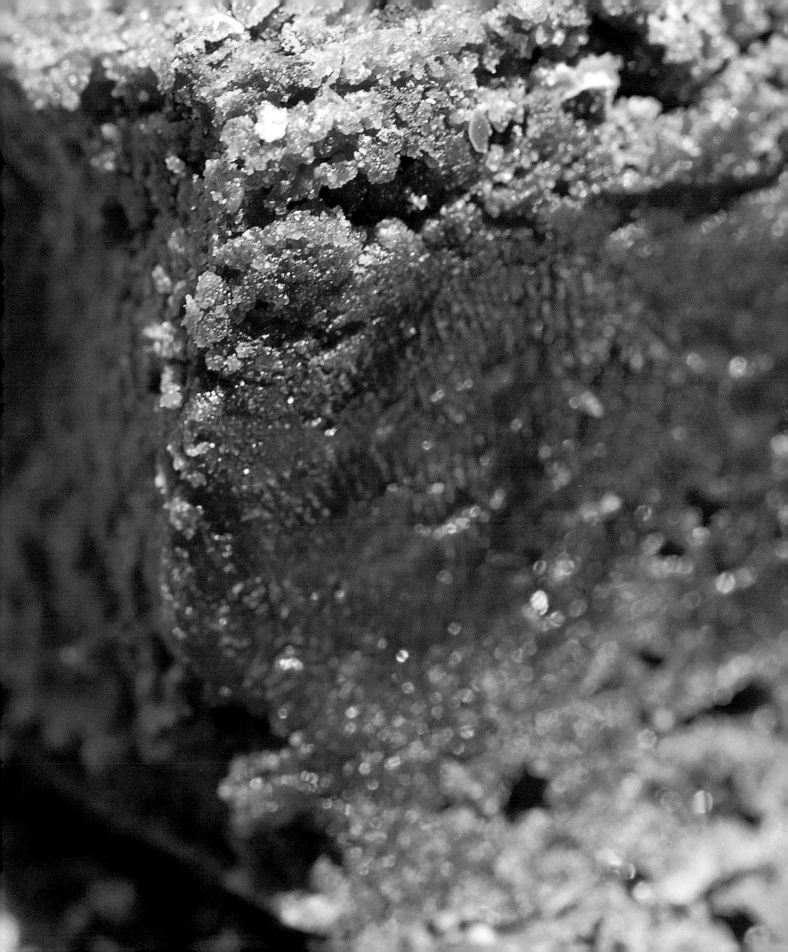

CHOCOLATE ALMOND BROWNIES

This recipe is flour-free, which makes it much richer. It is much more like a mousse than a conventional brownie, in the sense that it is absolutely riddled with chocolate flavour. So if you happen to be a chocoholic you will adore it. I serve it with faux whipped cream, although if you're not worried about dairy products you can always use cream itself sprinkled with toasted flaked almonds. I think you'll love it.

WHAT YOU NEED

400 g (14 oz) dark organic chocolate
200 g (7 oz) unsalted butter
8 eggs, separated
175 ml (6 fl oz) golden granulated sugar
3 tbsp finely ground almonds
2 tsp vanilla extract
200 g (7 oz) toasted almond flakes
small quantity shaved dark chocolate

HERE'S HOW

Preheat the oven to 180°C/350°F/Gas Mark 4. Use butter to grease the sides and bottom of a loose-bottomed 20-cm (8-in) square or round pan. Line the pan with greaseproof or waxed paper and grease the paper with butter as well. Now wrap the outside of the pan with aluminium foil.

Melt the chocolate and the butter, continuously stirring, in the top of a bain-marie until smooth and melted. Remove from the heat and let cool, stirring frequently. Using a food processor or electric mixer, beat the egg yolks and 6 tablespoons of sugar in a big bowl for about 3 minutes until pale and thick. Now very gently fold the chocolate mixture into the egg yolk one.

Beat the egg whites in a different large bowl to soft-peak stage. Slowly add the rest of the sugar and continue beating until peaks start to go firm. Fold the white into the chocolate mixture little by little. Pour the mixture into the pan and bake until the top puffs up and cracks and until a toothpick stuck into the middle comes out with some moist crumbs attached. This usually takes about 45 minutes. Remove from the oven and cool in the pan on a rack. Don't be distressed if the brownie mix 'falls': this is what is supposed to happen and what

gives it its rich flavour.

When it is cool, cut around the sides of the pan to loosen the brownies and invert the brownies on to a plate. Peel off the paper and cut into squares or slices. Serve with a sprinkle of slivered toasted almonds and shaved plain chocolate on top or add some fresh strawberries or Rose Petal and Ginger Couli **(see page 104)** made with raspberries.

ESPRESSO SORBET

serves 2

Long ago chocolate gained its reputation as a sexual stimulant. But coffee too holds many sexual secrets. This is why temperance organizations throughout the ages have campaigned vigorously against coffee as well as alcohol, speaking at length about its aphrodisiac qualities. My favourite form of coffee for love is iced espresso. I love the contrast of the intense coffee with the lightness of drinking it in - or spooning it out of - chilled glasses. It's not only good in the afternoon but makes a great treat in the garden on a sultry summer evening.

WHAT YOU NEED
90 ml (6 tbsp) strong black
  coffee
125 ml (4 fl oz) soya milk
crushed ice
honey to taste

HERE'S HOW
Pour the freshly brewed espresso and the soya milk into a powerful food processor with crushed ice. Blend well, but make sure you still maintain the icy quality of the drink so that you can serve it with a spoon. Pour into well-chilled, beautiful small glasses and drink immediately.

HIGHER TEA

There is something magic about the ritual of tea in every country in the world in which it is celebrated. Tea time is a moment to pause for relaxation and renewal, a time to enjoy the warmth of a fire in the dark of winter while munching on something delicious or to sit beneath the shade of a tree in the summer garden. Like any ritual, unless it's continually infused with new life, it can lose its sparkle and its meaning. For some time I wondered how to take the ritual of high tea - replete with finger foods - into the next century. Could watercress sandwiches not be born again in new form? What would happen if some of the conventional foods served at high tea were replaced by others? I began to play with adding sashimi and a delicious baked garlic spread to the list of simple-to-prepare delicious possibilities followed by sesame sticks and a beautiful little fruit jellies with whipped topping. Thus did higher tea come into being. It is unconventional and uncompromisingly delicious -

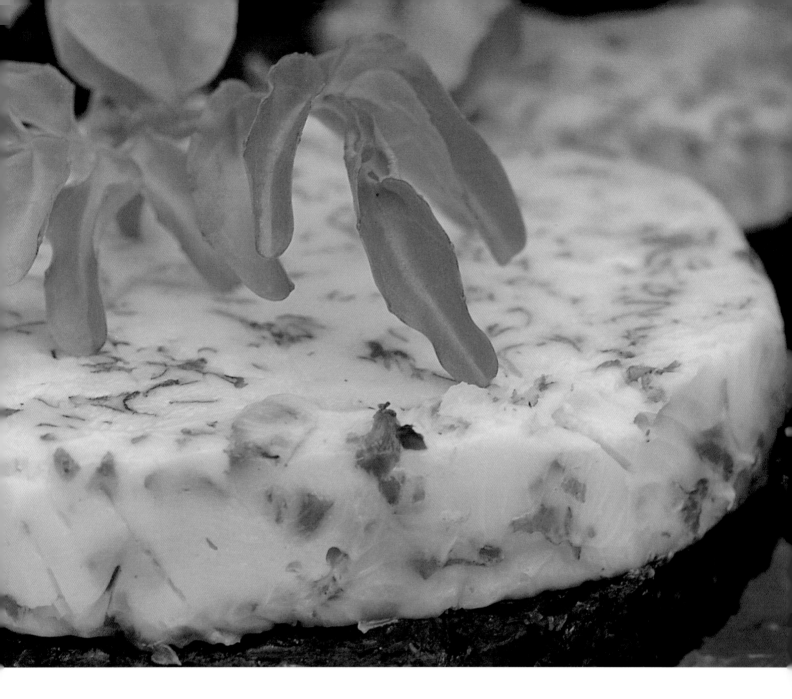

EVEN IF IT DOES COME AS A BIT OF

A SHOCK

TO DEAR OLD AUNTIE BECKY.

WATERCRESS TO GO

I use watercress with just about everything from potatoes to baked vegetables such as parsnips, beetroot, red and yellow peppers. I think it goes beautifully with oranges, lemons, grapes and pears in fruit salads. I've even been known to chop it finely and sprinkle it over fruit coulis, both for its colour and because its bitter flavour counteracts the sweetness.

Bitter-sweet

In Northern countries, watercress has grown wild for hundreds of years at the edges of free-flowing streams. Sadly, this delicious water-loving plant is no longer something you want to gather wild unless you're sure of the purity of the water in which it grows. Increased pollution in our waters and the possibility of stagnation increases the risk of liver fluke and of toxicity in the plant.

There is something wondrous about bitter green leaves like watercress. The Romans believed that eating them created a sensation of prickly nostrils, which in turn brought about a burst of vitality. In fact, their experience of this sensation, which came as a result of eating watercress, was so great that they named this green vegetable nasturtium, which in Latin means 'torment of the nose'. The name has long remained. The official name for the kind of watercress we use to make sandwiches is *Nasturtium officinale*.

Watercress makes great soup. Even putting it to boil in a good soup stock with some potatoes, lots of garlic and a bit of olive oil, then puréeing the lot makes a soup to delight everyone.

Watercress salads too are delicious. I like nothing better than to use watercress itself as a salad on its own. I don't even bother to tear off the leaves. I use the stems as well, served with a vinaigrette dressing and freshly slivered Parmesan on top, with lots of freshly ground red peppercorns and some Maldon sea salt. Like red mustard, mustard leaf, rocket and wild rocket, watercress adds a hot, tangy quality to almost anything you serve it with.

makes 4-12 sandwiches

WATERCRESS SANDWICHES

When it comes to high tea, watercress sandwiches are just about as traditional as you can get (see the picture on page 115). And little wonder, for watercress is one of Europe's oldest salad stuffs. Even the Greek playwright Aristophanes wrote about watercress, insisting that it carries strength and courage in its nature, and anyone who eats it can draw on these two virtues. In biblical times, watercress was considered one of the bitter herbs of the Passover - used to remind the Jews of their time of enslavement.

What could be more traditional for higher tea than watercress sandwiches? Maybe part of the reason for this is not only watercress's stimulating properties, but the fact that it goes with just about anything from avocados and cucumbers to potatoes, cheeses and anchovies - even pears, apples and plums do well garnished with watercress. I like to make my watercress sandwiches on very thin pumpernickel bread. They are far more delicious than the usual over-processed, floppy white that is traditionally used for making tea sandwiches.

WHAT YOU NEED
1/2 bunch of finely chopped watercress
50 g (2 oz) salted butter
4 slices of pumpernickel bread

HERE'S HOW
Put the watercress and softened butter into a food processor and blend. Remove and roll into a cylindrical shape inside a piece of greaseproof paper. Place in the refrigerator to chill. Once chilled, open it up and slice into pats. To serve, spread them on large pieces of pumpernickel bread or serve one pat per small round of pumpernickel. You can use this watercress butter over fish, grilled meat or vegetables - even mashed potatoes too. It's absolutely delicious.

SECRETS OF SASHIMI

Delightful summer or winter served with a cup of oolong, sencha or green Assam tea, is a plate of bright coloured sashimi. It is not only beautiful to look at but when it comes to fish there is no better way of eating it than raw, assuming the source of fish is a good one – absolutely fresh and caught in unpolluted waters. If ever you buy a fish fresh whole, make sure that its eyes are clear, never cloudy. The skin should look bright and shiny and it should bounce back when you touch it. Fish must never smell fishy. It needs to have just the faintest fragrance of the sea about it. Alternatively, there are a growing number of excellent organic food emporia that are extremely careful about the fish that they sell.

Flash freezing

To make absolutely sure that the fish is parasite-free – although I do believe that this compromises the texture and the flavour – you can always flash freeze it from 24 to 48 hours or freeze it in an ordinary freezer for a week then thaw, slice and serve immediately. In 1990, the Food and Drug Administration in the United States recommended that any fish served raw be blast-frozen to -35°C (-31°F) for 15 hours, or frozen by ordinary methods to -23°C (-10°C) for seven days before thawing and eating. If I'm going to freeze it (which I rarely do), I like to cut my fish into portions of about 150 g (5 oz) each so that when I'm ready to prepare the sashimi, the slicing of it is a simple task. When eating sashimi as a main course you need about 100-150 g (4-5 oz) of fish per person. If eating it as a starter or a small meal you need about half that amount.

I make my sashimi out of two or three kinds of fish at one time. Among the fish I particularly like are wild salmon, tuna – especially the huge, red tuna – squid (I use the body, rather than the tentacles), large white fish such as sea bass or groper, terakihi, sole, scallops and even crayfish or lobster (which makes some of the most delicious sashimi in the world).

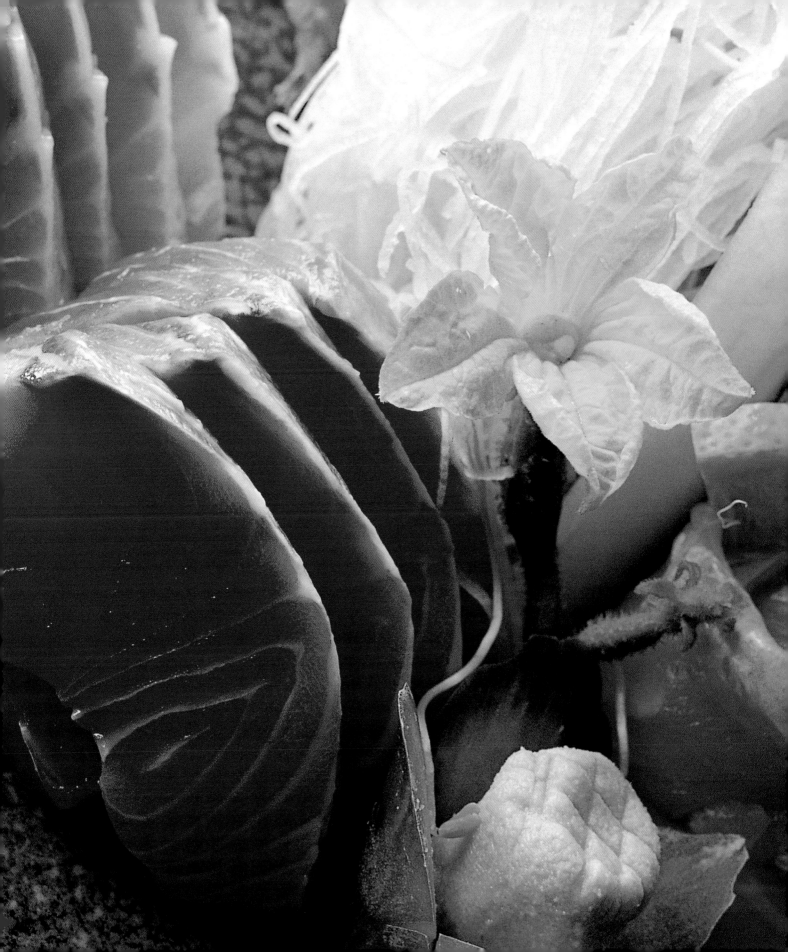

SASHIMI WITH DIPPING SAUCE

serves 4

WHAT YOU NEED
4 tbsp sake
125 ml (4 fl oz) mirin
5 cm (2 in) piece of kombu
125 ml (4 fl oz) tamari
2.5 cm (1 in) piece of fresh
  ginger, finely grated
10 g (1/4 oz) Bonita flakes

75-150 g (3-5 oz) mixed fresh
  fish per person
thick cucumber slices
a little thinly sliced gari
  (pickled ginger)
4 chrysanthemum leaves
  (optional)
1 tsp wasabe horseradish per
  person
40 g (1 1/2 oz) daikon (white
  radish), finely julienned
1/2 a lemon, sliced
parsley leaves to garnish

HERE'S HOW
Don't let the skill of the
Japanese chef put you off
making sashimi. What you need
is a very sharp knife and a
simple flat dish on which to
arrange things.

First make the dipping
sauce. Heat gently together the
sake and the mirin, then light
it to burn off any excess
alcohol. Add the kombu, tamari,
ginger and the loose Bonita
flakes. Bring to the boil and
simmer gently for 3 minutes.
Remove from the heat and pop
into the refrigerator if you
can for a few hours so that
the flavour develops.

For the sashimi, cut three
or four 9-mm (3/8-in) thick
slices of each of the fishes.
Arrange them on individual
dishes nestled into each other
with cucumber and gari slices
and maybe a chrysanthemum leaf.
Serve with wasabe horseradish,
daikon and some lemon and
parsley leaves accompanied by
small bowls of the dipping
sauce. Using chopsticks, dip
the fish and some daikon in a
little wasabe and then in the
dipping sauce.

SESAME STICKS

It's not easy to find yummy sweet treats that don't contain
wheat. Almost all the biscuits, cookies and bars available are
choc full of wheat flour. Sesame sticks fit the bill perfectly.
These delicious sweets are great to go with afternoon tea. They
are high in calcium and phosphorus as well as important essential
fatty acids. They are also easy to make and to turn into little
cookies – if you choose to drop them from your spoon.
Alternatively, if you choose to put them in a baking tin and
smooth them out to 12 mm (1/2 in) thick then bake them, you can
cut them into long sticks. Personally I like the sticks best. The
trick of making these sesame treats work is to make sure that you
leave them in the oven long enough to get the surface golden-
brown, so that when they cool they go ultra-crunchy. If you can't
find the almond or cashew butter listed in the ingredients, you
can use peanut, but it's nowhere near as good.

WHAT YOU NEED
500 g (1 lb 2 oz) raw,
    unbleached sesame seeds
100 g (4 oz) finely shredded
    coconut
50 g (2 oz) chopped almonds
4 tbsp almond butter or cashew
    butter
8 tbsp liquid honey
1/2 tsp salt
zest of 1 lemon, finely
    shredded
100 g (4 oz) golden granulated
    sugar or date sugar

HERE'S HOW
Preheat the oven to
150°C/300°F/Gas 2. Mix all of
the ingredients together and
then, if you choose to make
the sticks, smooth them out to
12 mm (1/2 in) thick on a
greased baking tin. Bake for 20
to 30 minutes. Remove from the
oven and cut into fingers while
still hot. The other way of
making them is to drop them
from a spoon, making small
cookies, and bake them that
way. Do be careful because
these will tend to stick
together once they're cold.

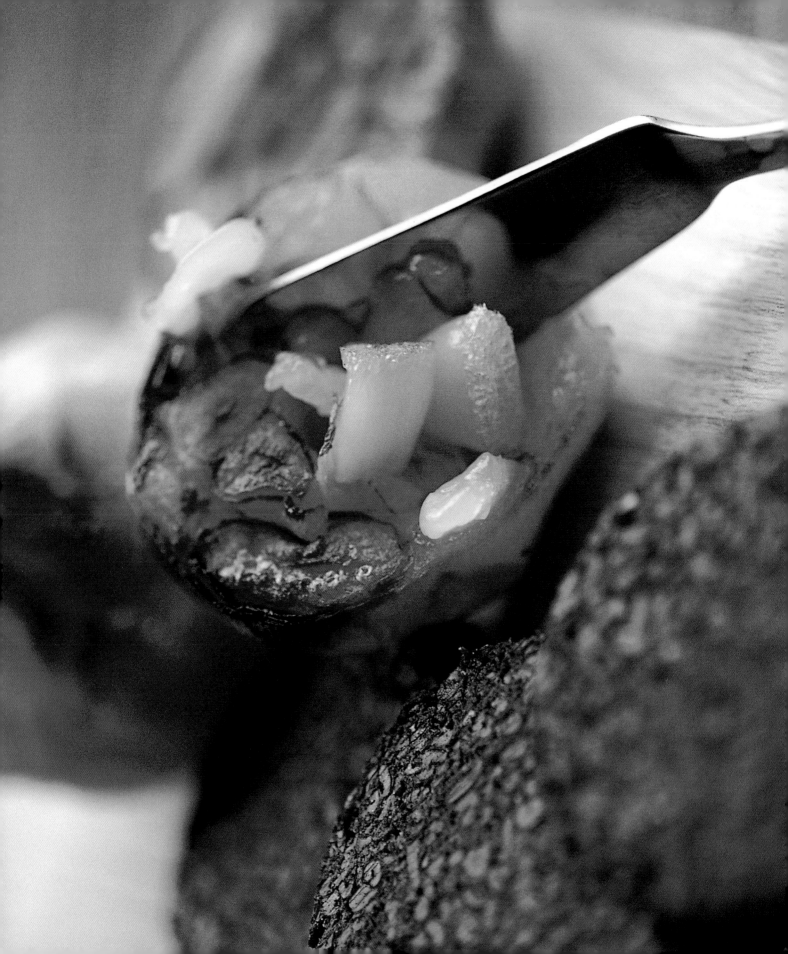

GET INTO GARLIC

These days, people take more garlic as a supplement than any other plant product except echinacea and ginseng. You see it promoted everywhere in advertisements that extoll its benefits. These are many. Garlic contains more than 200 different known plant chemicals, most of which have positive effects on the body - preventing illness, suppressing cancer cell growth and counteracting heart disease. So far there are more than 2,400 scientific studies on the health-promoting capacities of garlic and its main benefits are given. (For the Inside Story on garlic, see page 90.)

serves 8

BAKED GARLIC SPREAD

This is one of the most delicious spreads for home-baked bread that you'll ever find. It's low in fat and you can use it just as you use butter. It's wonderful for tea or as an addition to any meal.

WHAT YOU NEED
8 large whole garlic bulbs
3 tbsp extra-virgin olive oil
1 tsp Maldon sea salt and
   freshly ground pepper
parsley (optional)
basil (optional)

HERE'S HOW
Cut the whole garlics in half horizontally. Place cut side up on a baking sheet. Brush the cut side with olive oil. Bake at 200°C/400°F/Gas Mark 6 for 15 to 20 minutes - just until the cut surface browns and goes soft. Now sprinkle with salt and pepper. Serve as is, hot or cold on a plate with a butter knife for spreading.

GRAINS OF TRUTH

Forget the soft white bread made from refined wheat flour. There are better ways to go. Try Lavender Muffins (see page 36) as a vehicle for delicious spreads at tea, or rye crackers which impart crunchy texture and great flavour when spread with a fresh pesto. Grains come in tremendous variety, from wheat, oats, rye and barley to the more exotic varieties such as kamut and spelt (very close to the original wheat) and quinoa. (For the Inside Story on grains, see page 88.)

TOFU SANDWICH ON RYE

Wholegrain rye is a great vehicle for any hearty sandwich – the kind you eat at tea that will carry you all the way through the evening without hunger. Here I have taken teppan yaki grilled tofu slices, added some alfalfa sprouts and sliced yellow tomatoes with a leaf or two of lettuce from the garden and placed it all between dark rye bread that has been spread with a garlic aïoli (see page 178). I topped it off with a few tiny leaves of fresh basil and served it on a simple wooden tray with a tall glass of chilled summer cooler.

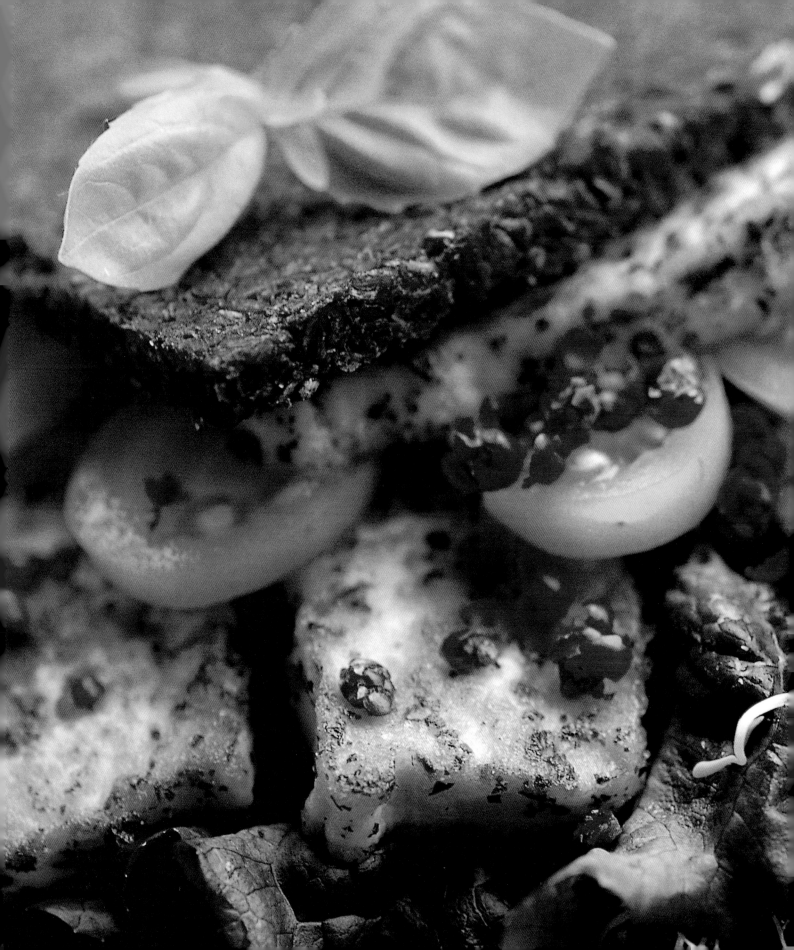

GELS AND JELLIES

Jellies or gels made with agar agar are not only delicious and natural - they often need no extra sweetening to make them work. They are also good for you and very easy to make. Agar agar makes a firmer gel than ordinary gelatine gels, which makes it great for picnics and garden parties. You can prepare simple jellies by liquidizing fruit such as raspberries, strawberries, seedless grapes or plums in a food processor and then straining.

It's all in the quantity

You can buy agar agar in Oriental shops or good health food stores. It comes either in powder, flakes or kanten bars. You can use it to make wonderful jams and toppings that are as sweet or unsweet as you like, as well as fruit jellies and even moulded salads. Generally speaking, a 1/4 teaspoon of agar agar powder is equal to 3 tablespoons of the light flakes or 1 kanten bar, and out of this quantity you will be able to gel about 450 ml (16 fl oz) of liquid.

If you want a firmer gel, as in making a jelly to mould and then turn out, use a little more agar agar. If you want a light jelly that is soft, quivering and barely set - the kind that you serve in tall champagne glasses and which slides off the teaspoon - use less. Experiment until you get just the right consistency for your purposes. (For the Inside Story on agar agar, see page 93.)

FRUIT GELS

serves 6

This is my recipe for a firm agar agar fruit gel. You can serve it as a gel fruit salad, a rich dessert or, by replacing the fruit juice with a vegetable broth and adding grated carrots, sprouts and seaweed, avocado and some chopped onions, create a moulded vegetable salad instead of a fruit dish.

WHAT YOU NEED

450 ml (16 fl oz) chopped
    fresh fruit, e.g. mangoes,
    papayas, passion fruit,
    apples, mandarins, grapes,
    berries
8 tbsp raw honey
3-4 tbsp agar agar flakes
900 ml (32 fl oz) grape,
    pineapple, orange or apple
    juice
zest of 1 lemon, finely
    shredded (optional)
2 tbsp fresh lemon juice
1 tsp vanilla extract

HERE'S HOW

Cover the bottom of a glass
mould with fruit and sweeten
with honey. Mix the agar agar
with 250 ml (8 fl oz) of the
fruit juice. Let it sit while
heating the remaining juice.
Add to the heated fruit juice
and stir, simmering for 2
minutes. Cool. Add the lemon
zest, fresh lemon juice and
vanilla extract. Mix well. Pour
the gel over the fruit and let
it sit in the refrigerator.
Just before serving, turn the
jelly out of the mould and
serve in slices with Light
Whipped Topping **(see page 182)**.

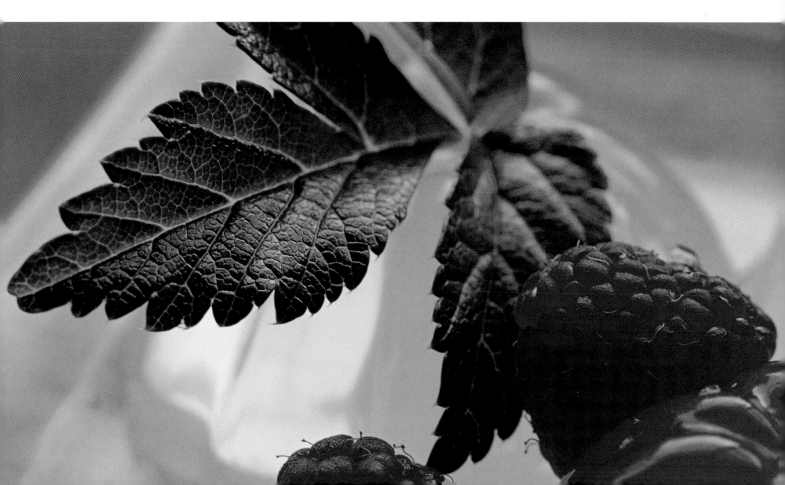

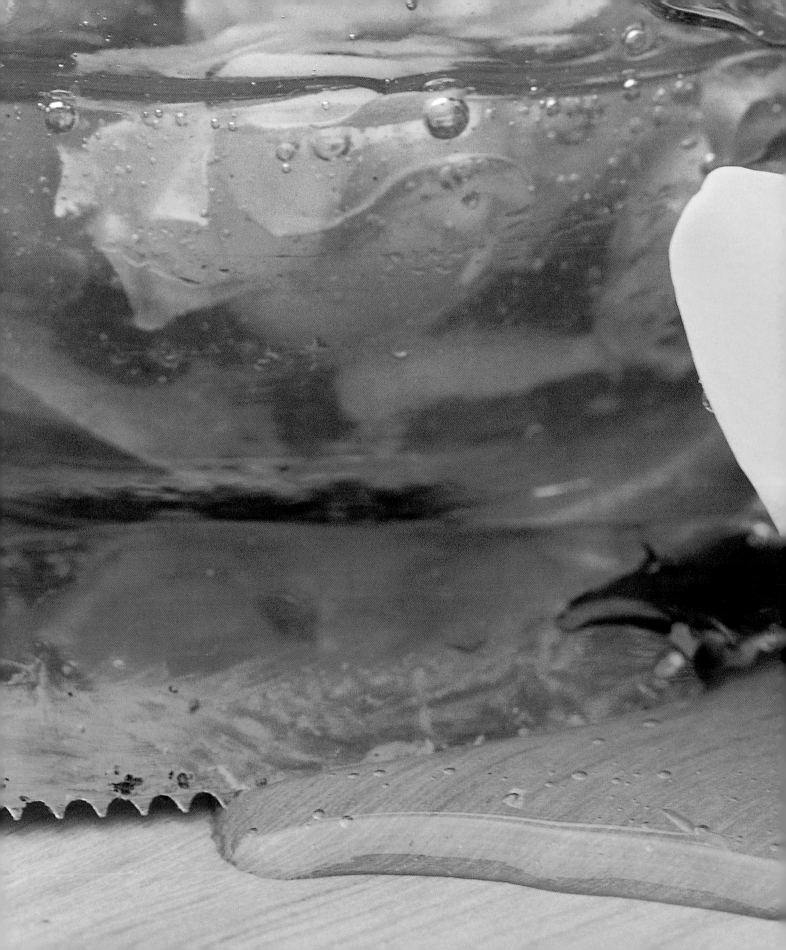

makes 500 g (1 lb 2 oz)

FLOWER HONEY

I adore honey. As a result I have tried just about every kind in the world. Some honeys, such as acacia, are light and fine. They never go solid; however, they are not very useful in cooking because they tend to lose their flavour. Others, such as tupelo or manuka, are very strong-flavoured, which tends to remain even when cooked. Of all the honeys in the world, the ones I like best are those to which flowers have been added. Not only are flower honeys beautiful to serve at high tea, they are fun to make. You can create them using whatever flowers you happen to have available in the garden. The flowers I suggest are lavender, jasmine, red clover, scented geranium or rose. If the flowers are very small, like lavender, they need not be chopped. Just remove them from their stems and throw the stems away.

WHAT YOU NEED
2 handfuls fresh flower petals
500 g (1 lb 2 oz) honey

HERE'S HOW
Put the flower petals and the honey into a bain-marie and gently heat over boiling water for 5 to 10 minutes. Take the mixture off and pour it back into its jar. Let cool. Cover it and let it sit for two weeks to absorb the flavour of the flowers. Now it's ready to use, either strained or as is – flowers and all.

SUMMER COOLERS

ORANGE GINGER BEER

Based on the traditional recipe for ginger beer, this is one great drink for higher tea. You can have it as is or you can mix a little fizzy water with it. Sometimes I use only half a litre (16 fl oz) of water instead of a full litre (1 3/4 pints) when making the recipe, then top up just before serving with half a litre (16 fl oz) of sparkling water. This recipe will keep for four or five days in the refrigerator. (For the Inside Story on ginger, see page 92.)

WHAT YOU NEED

50-100 g (2-4 oz) piece of fresh ginger, roughly chopped

1 litre (1 3/4 pints) spring water

250 ml (8 fl oz) acacia honey (you can use another liquid honey if you prefer, but acacia has such a fine flavour that I like it best)

250 ml (8 fl oz) freshly squeezed orange juice

1 tbsp finely shredded orange zest

1/2 tsp ground cinnamon

HERE'S HOW

Place the roughly chopped ginger and the water in a food processor. Add the acacia honey, orange juice, orange zest and the cinnamon and blend. Stir well and put in the refrigerator for 24 hours so the flavours meld. Strain, then chill for another hour. Pour over ice to serve immediately.

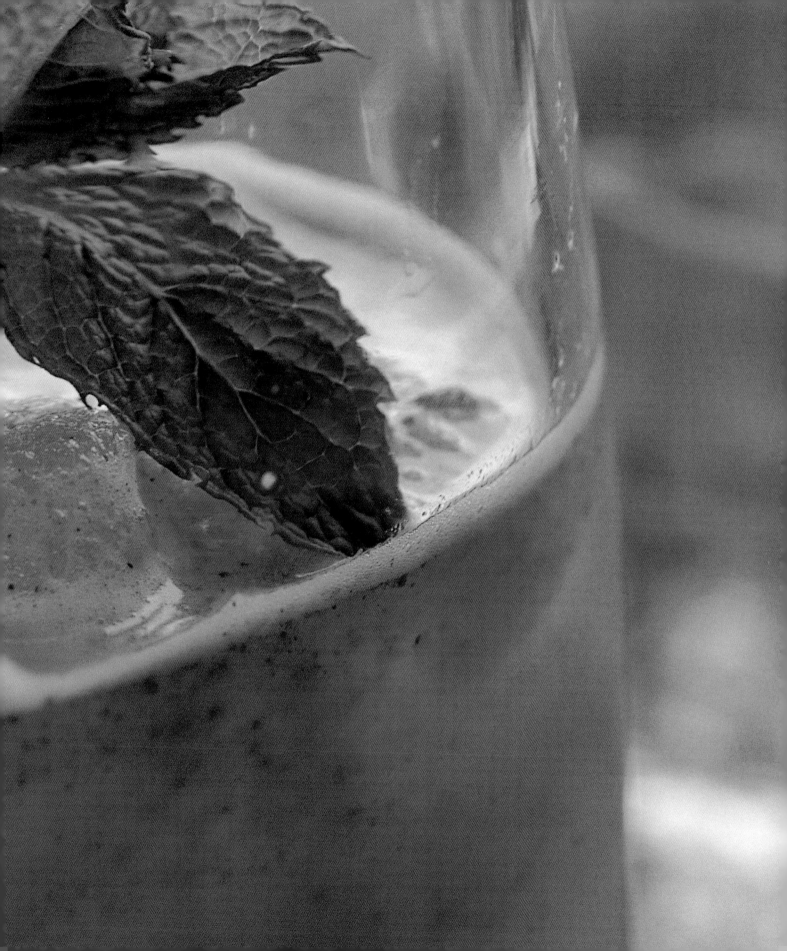

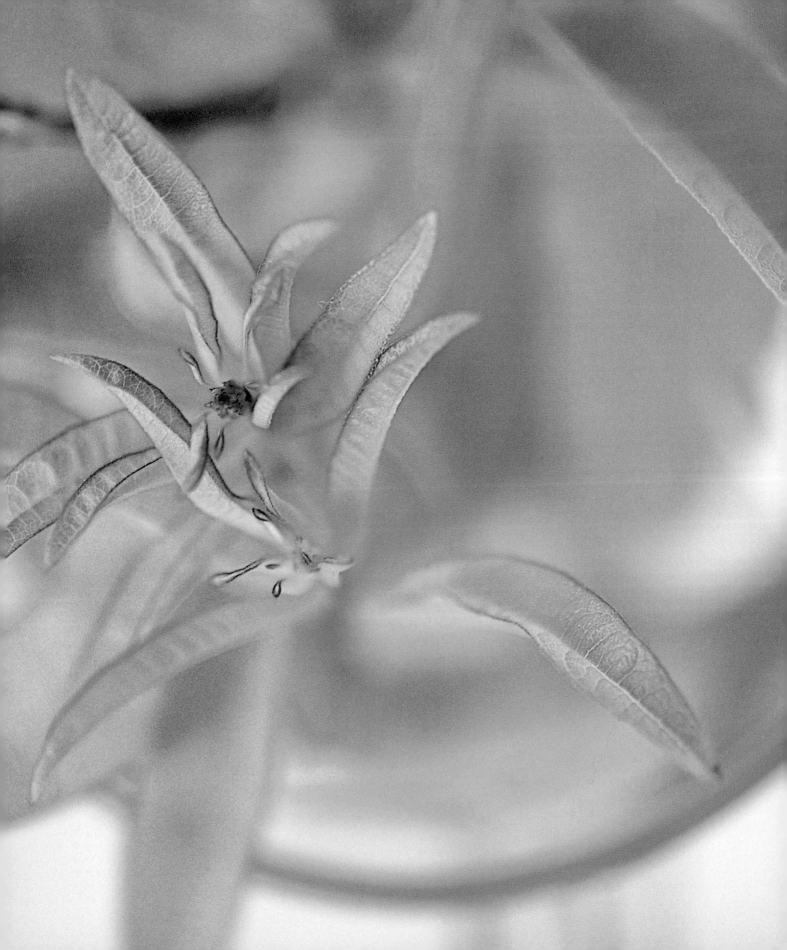

SPIKY LEMON TEA

This recipe is made with one of my all time favourite green-tasting herbs – lemon verbena. Lemon verbena tea shares the slight spikiness of the plant which has many health-giving properties. It helps combat nausea and stomach upsets. It is also useful to clear colds and fevers. Recent research shows that this plant has both antibacterial and anti-viral properties. The parts you use for tea are the leaves and, if you have them, the flowering tops, which should be harvested just when they're beginning to open. They will freeze well for future use.

The lemon verbena plant has a strong lemony flavour, which goes beautifully with lemon juice. Lemon itself, like all citrus fruits, helps to balance our Western diet, where we get excessive sodium, by supplying its antagonist, potassium. This makes it useful in keeping blood pressure at a healthy level. Finally, the humble lemon has such a beautiful flavour that I use both the juice and the zest in many dishes that I prepare.

WHAT YOU NEED
about 18 lemon verbena leaves
   with the flowering tops or
   4 tsp dried leaves of lemon
   verbena
juice of 1 lemon
liquid honey to taste
   (optional)
lemon verbena leaves or lemon
   zest to garnish

HERE'S HOW
Infuse the lemon verbena leaves for 5 minutes in a teapot covered with boiling water. Add the lemon juice and sweetener to taste. It's actually very refreshing with no sweetener but if you feel you must, then go for tupelo or manuka honey because of their intense flavours. Garnish and serve immediately.

POWER FOODS

8

The word 'protein' quite literally means 'primary substance'. It is an appropriate name. For every tissue in your body from your brain to your little fingernail is built of and repaired with protein. Amino acids, the building blocks of protein, are both central factors in most of the processes of the body too – like making antibodies against infection, creating hormones and overall strength. Grill fish and meat teppan yaki style, bake them in paper or banana leaves, slow roast chicken, game or turkey, and serve them with a surprising rosemary and white wine sorbet. However you prepare them,

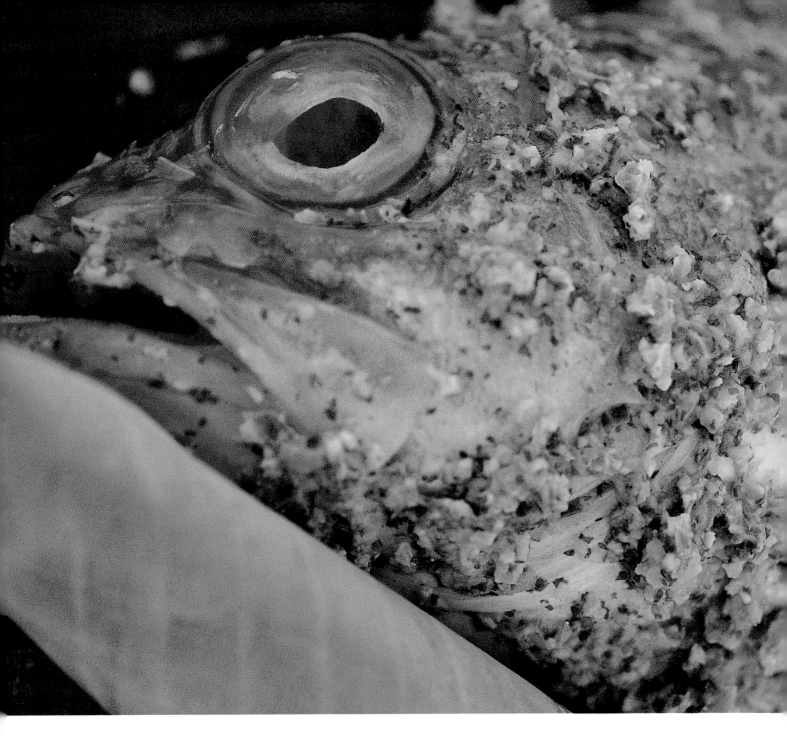

POWER FOODS HOLD THE CENTRE OF EVERY
IMPORTANT MEAL.

TEPPAN YAKI COMES TO BIRTH

I grew up on the West Coast of America very close to a traditional Japanese family who metaphorically adopted me as their fourth daughter. The father in the family was a Buddhist priest - later director of all the Japanese Buddhist churches in California. As a result, I was not only steeped in Japanese mythology and religion but also in traditions of food preparation. I learned to make sukiyaki, udon and any number of other Japanese dishes as part of my upbringing. I loved the long traditions behind home-made pickles and noodles, the wonderful methods of cooking rice and making vinegars.

A great Japanese tradition

In recent years I have spent much time in Japan developing natural health and beauty products and functional foods. One of the many characteristics of the Japanese culture which I adore is their relationship to tradition itself. Not only do they preserve so many splendid ancient methods of food preparation, marshal arts, gardening and meditation practices, they are also enormously innovative - continually evolving new methods of doing things which pave the way for new traditions to be born.

Teppan yaki is just such a new tradition. It is a way of cooking protein foods as well as vegetables that developed in the last thirty years in Japan, and which not only couldn't be healthier but is incredibly delicious. For teppan yaki sears into foods their intrinsic flavour and protects the integrity of their nutritional value. Foods like meat, fish, shellfish, chicken and game as well as vegetables like bok choy, bamboo shoots, sprouts and carrots are quickly grilled on a flat heated sheet. The ultimate in fast food preparation, it takes from 30 seconds to cook squid and 1 minute for scallops to 5 minutes for boneless chicken and 10 minutes for pork.

Ideally, you need a teppan yaki grill. Good ones are just beginning to come on the market. The best consist of stainless steel electric flat plates or aluminium treated with non-stick technology. They plug into the wall and can be used either on the kitchen work surface or directly on the table itself. Prepare the raw ingredients, such as spare ribs, prawns, tofu, or finely sliced steak plus the vegetables to go with them, by chopping them and placing them on a dish. Then you cook the food as you eat it, making sure never to overcook anything (this is easy to do when cooking teppan yaki since it cooks so quickly). Either eat the foods as is or serve with simple sauces, pestos or salsas. You can even skewer fish and vegetables and cook things this way.

If you don't have a teppan yaki grill, you can begin to experience the delights of this way of cooking using a heavy crêpe pan or even a large frying pan – electric or otherwise. But somehow these substitutes are never as good as the real thing. Once you get into teppan yaki food preparation, I predict you will want to buy an Oriental grill to make the whole process more graceful and simple. Many of the sauces in this book – from Basil Pesto **(page 181)** to the dipping sauces **on page 141** are ideal companions for teppan yaki grilled foods.

Which meats to use for teppan yaki grilled food

Beef: sirloin, rump, rib eye, fillet.

Chicken: breast fillet, thigh fillet.

Lamb: fillet, cutlets, sliced leg or shoulder.

Fish: fillets.

Shellfish: prawns in shells or shelled, mussels in shells, clams in shells, shelled scallops.

A TEPPAN YAKI FEAST

serves 4

The single most important nutritional feature of meat is its cellular structure, which is very similar to our own. This means that the nutrients absorbed from meat are very quickly and easily transformed into our tissue and blood. Consequently, small amounts of meat can be enormously strengthening to people who are deficient in strength and energy. This recipe allows for vegetarians who eat fish. (For the Inside Story on the meat question, see page 94.)

WHAT YOU NEED
500 g (1 lb 2 oz) pork, lamb, chicken breasts and beef sirloin cut into 6-12 mm (1/4-1/2 in) strips

or

500 g (1 lb 2 oz) prawns, scallops, squid, fish or tofu
1 tbsp sesame oil
500 g (1 lb 2 oz) raw fresh vegetables, e.g. bok choy, carrots, onions, spring onions, shallots, courgettes, sliced or shredded
garlic cloves, sliced
ginger, finely shredded
chillies, chopped (optional)
tamari to season (optional)
Maldon sea salt and freshly ground pepper
1-2 dipping sauces (optional)

HERE'S HOW
Heat the grill or pan to hot so that when you flick a few drops of water on the grill it jumps. Add sesame oil. (If you have a non-stick grill you don't even need the oil.) You can cook garlic slivers before placing other foods on the grill to add flavour. Place the food on the grill and cook for the appropriate time:
Beef: 3-4 minutes each side
Pork: 4 minutes each side
Chicken slices: 2-3 minutes each side
Lamb: 2 minutes each side
Fish: 4-5 minutes each side
Scallops: 1 minute each side
Squid: 30 seconds each side
Prawns: 3 minutes each side
Vegetables: 2-3 minutes
Tofu: 3 minutes each side
Garlic, ginger, chillies: 3-5 minutes
Remove and serve immediately with dipping sauces.

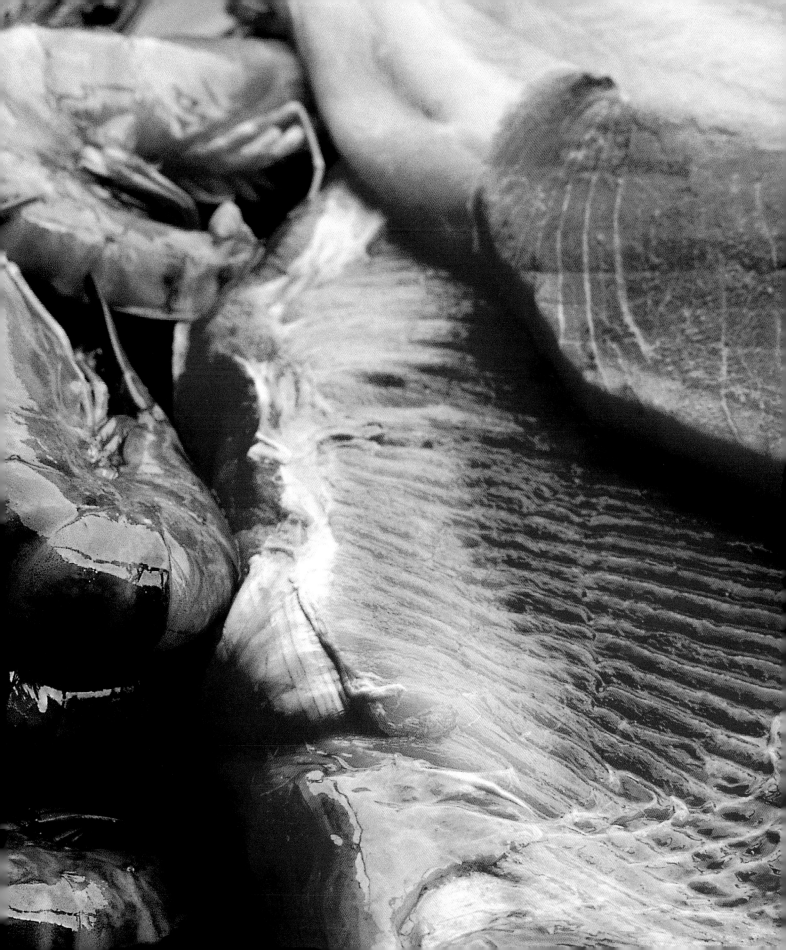

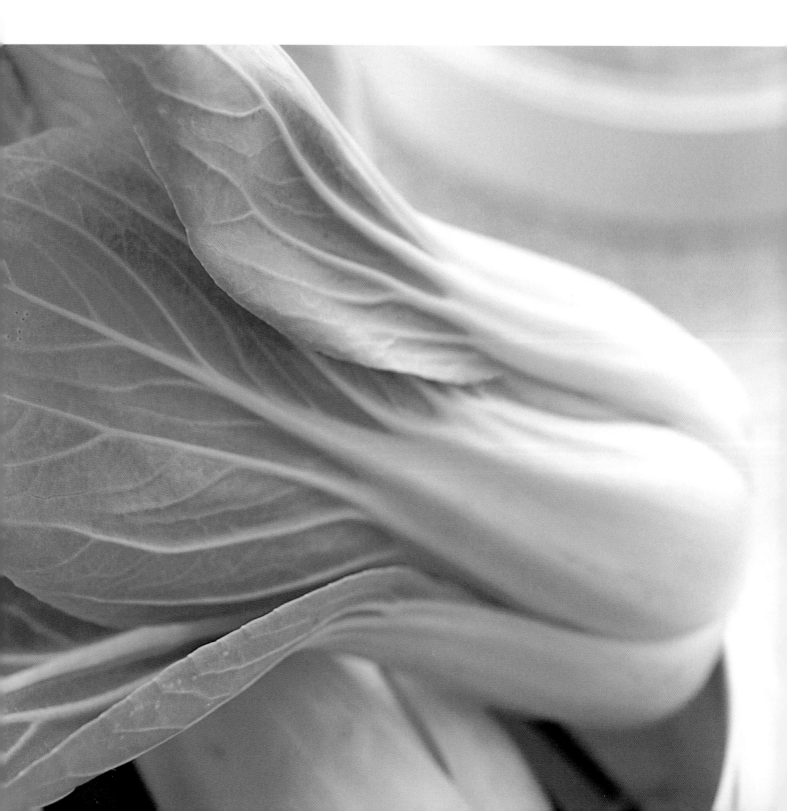

makes 250 ml (8 fl oz)

HONEY AND PINEAPPLE DIPPING SAUCE

WHAT YOU NEED

200 g (7 oz) fresh pineapple
2 garlic cloves, crushed
1-2 tbsp honey
1 tsp allspice
1 tsp freshly ground nutmeg
1 tsp ground cinnamon
1/4 tsp ground cloves
Maldon sea salt

HERE'S HOW

Mix together all the ingredients and let stand for 15 minutes. Then use as a marinade before cooking or as a dipping sauce afterwards. It is great for salmon, meat and chicken.

makes a small bowlful for dipping

LEMON AND RICE WINE DIPPING SAUCE

WHAT YOU NEED

125 ml (4 fl oz) lemon juice
2 garlic cloves, crushed
2 tbsp tamari
6 tbsp rice wine
Maldon sea salt

HERE'S HOW

Mix together all the ingredients and refrigerate until needed. This dipping sauce is good on seafood of all kinds.

makes 175 ml (6 fl oz)

SESAME MISO DIPPING SAUCE

WHAT YOU NEED

125 ml (4 fl oz) rice wine
3 tbsp golden granulated sugar
1 tbsp miso
2 tbsp sesame seeds, ground in a coffee grinder or food processor
1 garlic clove, crushed

HERE'S HOW

Combine all the ingredients. Can be served immediately. This one is ideal for vegetables.

CRUNCHY GREEN PRAWNS

serves 4

When it comes to prawns, green means raw. These are the best. You can buy them fresh or frozen in every form - shelled, unshelled, whole or heads removed. If you are lucky enough to find fresh ones, make sure they really are fresh since, like other shellfish, prawns go off fast. Plan to eat them the day you buy them. I love to eat them whole, partly because they are so beautiful and partly because I like the crunchy texture of the shells. I always eat the shells - usually not the heads unless they are very small. (For the Inside Story on prawns, see page 93.)

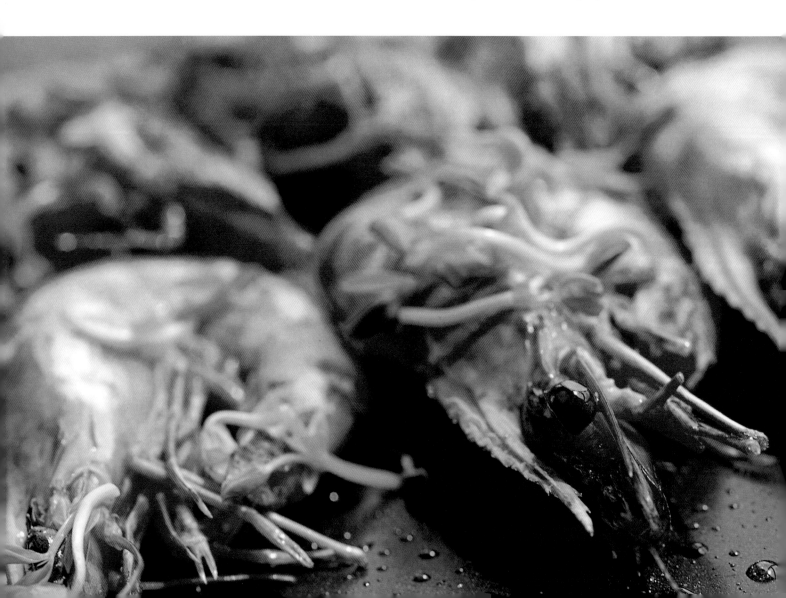

WHAT YOU NEED

750 g (1 lb 10 oz) King
  prawns, uncooked, and peeled
  and
  de-veined if you wish
2 limes, cut in wedges
2 tbsp fresh coriander, chopped

FOR THE MARINADE

3-4 tbsp extra-virgin olive oil
1 tbsp spring onions, finely
  chopped
2.5 cm (1 in) piece of fresh
  ginger, finely shredded
small handful of fresh
  coriander, chopped
2 tbsp sake or dry sherry
freshly ground pepper
juice and finely shredded zest
  of 2 small limes or 1 lemon
5 garlic cloves, finely chopped
1/2 tsp mustard seeds, broken
  up with a mortar and pestle
mangetout sprout heads to use
  as a garnish (optional)

HERE'S HOW

Wash the prawns in cold water and then dry with a tea towel. Place all the ingredients for the marinade, except the lime zest, chopped garlic, mustard seeds and 1/4 of the chopped coriander, into a food processor. Purée to a paste. Pour into a bowl, add the remaining ingredients and mix into the paste by hand. Place the prawns in the bowl and turn them over and over until they are covered with the paste. Put on to a flat glass dish and cover. Set in a cool place for at least 3 hours.

Cook on a teppan yaki grill, a barbecue or under a grill in the oven until crunchy. Serve with lime wedges and coriander and don't throw away any of the remaining cooked or uncooked marinade. It is delicious to spread over the crunchy prawns. It takes only a couple of minutes a side to fry these and very little more under a hot grill or on a barbecue - all you want is for them to turn opaque. However you cook them, eat them with your fingers - shell and all. I serve these prawns with a combination of brown and wild rices - about half and half - and a bright green salad with wild rocket and whatever fresh herbs, from basil to lovage, that I can harvest from the garden or find at the market.

serves 4

SNAPPER IN BANANA LEAVES

This recipe calls for banana leaves - just because they are so
beautiful with the red snapper and because this is how I learned
to cook fish in the South Pacific. But paper will do just as well
if you can't come by the banana leaves. I use aluminium foil only
as a last resort. When you cook anything acid, such as a protein
food or a fruit like tomato, in aluminium it leaches some of the
metal into the food, and aluminium is something we are all better
off without. Don't feel that you have to use red snapper. Try
other types of fish, such as red mullet, John Dory or what looks
freshest when you are shopping.

When buying ginger, look for a firm ginger root. In truth,
ginger is not really a root at all. It is part of the stem of
this tropical plant, which happens to grow beneath the ground.
Make sure the ginger you buy has no mould on it. When you bring
it home keep it wrapped in a paper bag in the refrigerator. This
way it will stay fresh for several weeks. You can also freeze
ginger very easily. Another way you can keep it fresh is to seal
it in a tightly closed jar in the refrigerator.

WHAT YOU NEED FOR THE PASTE
3 green chillies, de-seeded and
  chopped
1 stalk of lemon grass, chopped
6 garlic cloves, peeled and
  finely chopped
1 onion, peeled and chopped
6 cm (2 1/4 in) piece of fresh
  ginger, chopped
25 g (1 oz) bunch coriander
  (root and all), chopped
15 g (1/2 oz) mint, chopped
zest of 1 lime, finely shredded
1 tsp ground roasted cumin
1 tsp fennel seeds, dry toasted
1/2 tsp freshly ground pepper

2 tbsp solid honey
juice of 2 limes
60 g (2 1/2 oz) unsweetened
  creamed coconut, grated

2 snappers (approximately
  500 g/1 lb 2 oz), cleaned,
  scaled and dorsal fins
  removed
banana leaves
greaseproof paper or aluminium
  foil
1 tbsp extra-virgin olive oil
limes

HERE'S HOW

Place all the paste ingredients in a food processor and purée. If the paste seems too thick, add a little warm water to get the right consistency so that it is moist and sticks together well. Wash and dry the fish and make a few diagonal slits through the skin on each side. Rub half the paste all over the fish, inside and out. Wrap in banana leaves, paper or aluminium foil to enclose the fish completely and secure with string. It is essential to create a really tight package so the juices don't escape while the fish is cooking. Refrigerate until you're ready to cook.

Heat the grill or oven to 200°C/400°F/Gas Mark 6. Rub the parcels all over with oil and grill or bake for about 8 to 10 minutes each side. In the oven it takes about 20 minutes. The outside leaves will char, but the fish inside will cook gently. Thin the remaining paste with 2 to 3 tablespoons of warm water if it is too stiff and serve with the fish and wedges of lime.

OTHER WAYS TO GO

Fast and easy: Fill a greaseproof paper parcel with fish, clams, prawns and scallops. Add some lemon juice, Oriental fish sauce, garlic and Cajun seasoning **(see page 43)** and bake in a hot oven for 5 to 8 minutes. Serve immediately.

Salt crust: This is a particularly good way of cooking salmon, though I would suggest baking it in the oven at 200°C/400°F/ Gas Mark 6 for about 20 minutes. Spread 500 g (1 lb 2 oz) of rock salt on a dish, lay the fish on this, then cover it with another 500 g (1 lb 2 oz) of salt and bake.

Simple seasoning: The fish can be seasoned with something as simple as fresh oregano, olive oil and the juice and zest of half a lemon for a faster, simpler meal.

Add vegetables: New potatoes wrapped individually in greaseproof paper and baked in the oven with the fish is a fun way of serving vegetables.

serves 4

CORIANDER TOFU

Thanks to the intense flavour of coriander, this herb works well to enhance the bland flavour of tofu. This recipe goes particularly well with steamed vegetables - especially broccoli - and brown rice. Or make a tofu sandwich of it, or add this tofu to a salad to make it a one-bowl meal rich in protein and in plant factors for health.

WHAT YOU NEED
400 g (14 oz) firm tofu
2 tbsp extra-virgin olive oil
  or sesame oil
5 cm (2 in) piece of fresh
  ginger, finely shredded
handful fresh coriander, finely
  chopped
1 tbsp tamari
1 tsp honey
Maldon sea salt and freshly
  ground red peppercorns

HERE'S HOW
Cut the tofu crosswise into slices that are approximately 9 mm (3/8 in) thick. Mix together all the other ingredients in a bowl, then dip each tofu slice into the mixture you have created. Heat a heavy frying pan, grill or teppan yaki grill **(see page 136)**. Spray just enough olive oil on top of the grill so the tofu will not stick. Place the tofu on the grill, sprinkle with Maldon sea salt and freshly ground red peppercorns and cook at a high temperature until browned. Turn and brown again. Serve immediately as a tofu sandwich or in a tofu salad or simply as is with loads of beautifully coloured fresh vegetables. The whole process of cooking takes no more than 3 to 5 minutes.

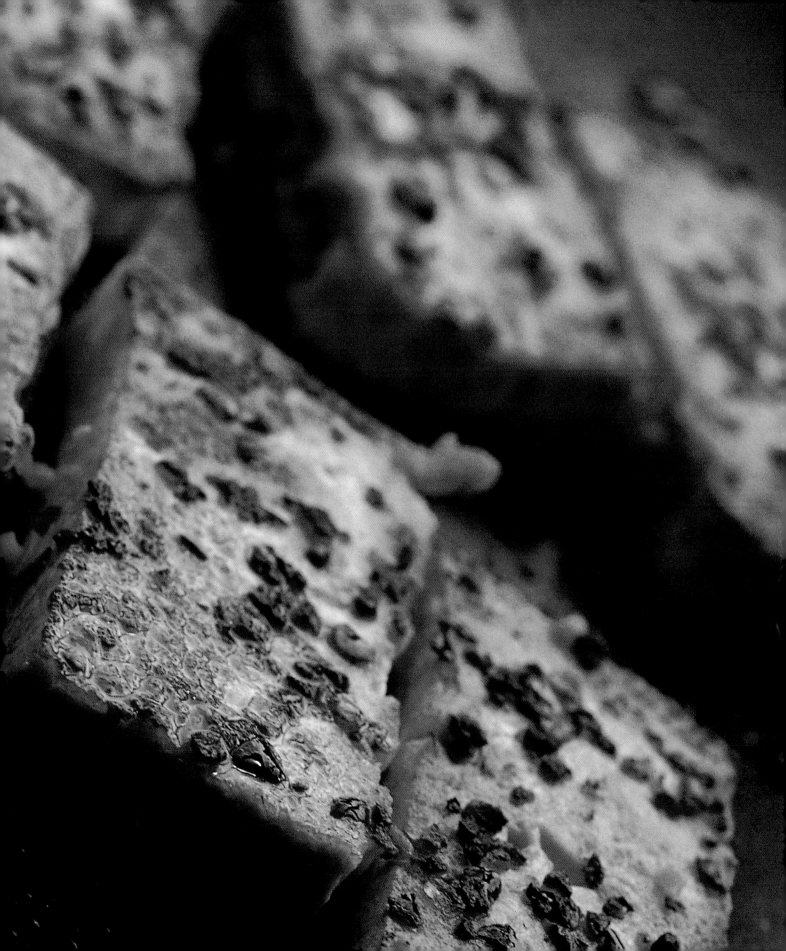

SAGE SLASHED CHICKEN

Unless I am in a great hurry or feeling unusually lazy, I never put any roast in the oven without first infusing it with whatever fresh herbs I have on hand. In the case of lamb it is often rosemary and garlic. For duck or game birds it is usually thyme and for chicken, sage. After cleaning the bird, I make slashes with a sharp knife into the thighs and legs, breast and back. Then I stuff them with leaves of fresh sage and sometimes garlic so that the leaves lie beneath the surface of the skin making beautiful patterns in the finished roast. The result is a dish filled with flavour that has been drawn right into the meat – not only beautiful to look at but delicious to eat.

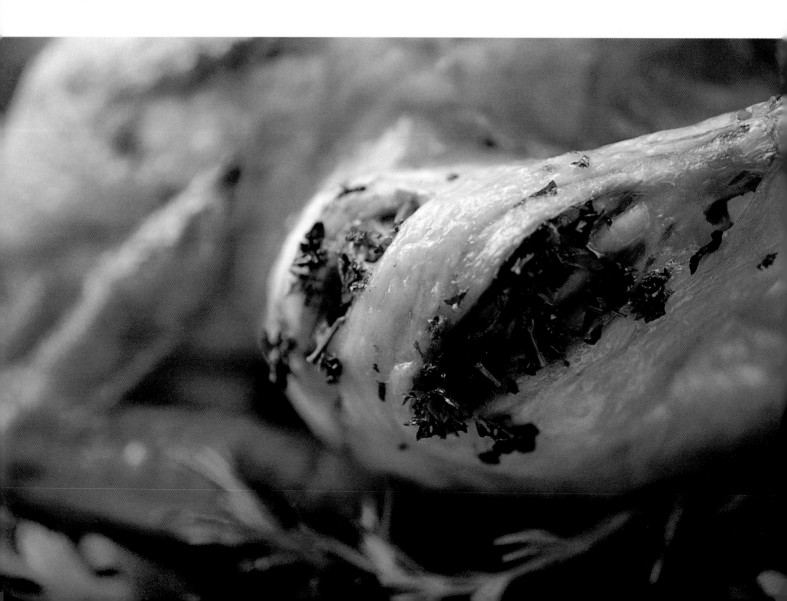

MARJORAM HONEYED QUAIL

These little members of the pheasant family are easy to prepare and a delight to eat. I like to cook them for small dinner parties as they take very little preparation yet taste so good. You need a good heavy pot with a lid, some fresh herbs from the garden and not a lot else. I use flower honey **(see page 129)** for this dish.

WHAT YOU NEED
4-6 quail
Maldon sea salt and freshly
    ground black pepper
plenty of sprigs of fresh
    marjoram
2 tbsp extra-virgin olive oil
1 tbsp fresh savory, chopped
725 g (1 lb 8 oz) tiny
    potatoes, scrubbed but not
    peeled
good handful of raisins
1 glass dry white wine
3 tbsp flower petal honey

HERE'S HOW
Wash and dry the quail and rub them inside and out with salt and pepper. Place a couple of sprigs of marjoram inside each. Heat the olive oil in the bottom of a heavy pan and put the quail in to brown, turning frequently. Remove from heat, add chopped savory, potatoes, raisins, white wine and honey as well as more sprigs of marjoram and bake for half an hour. Garnish with more marjoram and serve. These little birds are also delicious served cold later.

serves 6

ROSEMARY AND WHITE WINE GRANITA

Meat needs herbs and there is no better way to get them than by serving a herb-infused granita just after eating it. A cool, uplifting experience, this is a dish that you can serve with roast lamb, chicken and even baked fish, or in between courses to clear the palate. It also makes a surprising and very beautiful dessert. You can either make this dish in a tray in the freezer or you can use an ice-cream maker or sorbetière. (For the Inside Story on rosemary, see page 92.)

WHAT YOU NEED

1 tbsp chopped fresh rosemary
250 ml (8 fl oz) water
300-400 ml (10-14 fl oz) maple syrup, rice syrup or honey
250 ml (8 fl oz) dry white wine
2 tbsp lime juice
more fresh rosemary sprigs, preferably with flowers, as a garnish

HERE'S HOW

Put the rosemary into a saucepan with the water and maple syrup, rice syrup or honey and bring it to a slow boil. Take it off the heat and add the wine. Cool. Cover and then refrigerate overnight. Now add the lime juice and strain. If you have an ice-cream maker, make the granita in that. If not, put the mixture into a shallow tray in the freezer and turn down the temperature as far as possible. Let it remain until the edges are hard but the centre is still watery. Mix the edges with the centre and put back into the freezer. Repeat until granita is set but not rock hard. Scrape into a processor and mix quickly, just enough to soften the pointed crystals. Place in a serving dish and pop into the freezer for another 15 minutes.

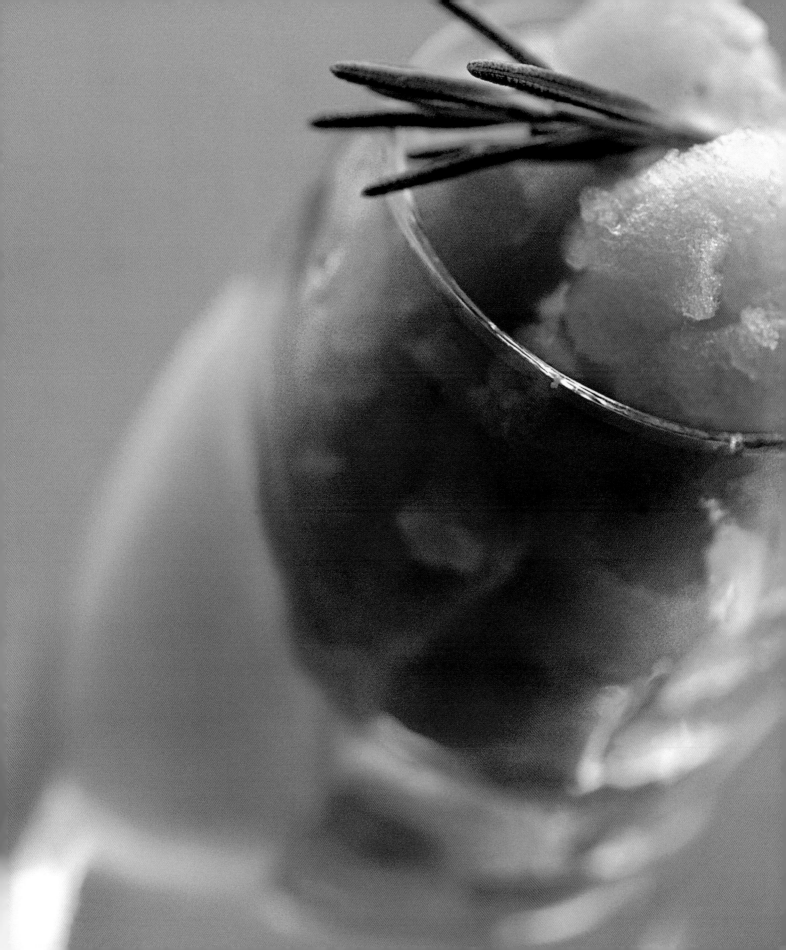

GO BRIGHT

I never met a vegetable I didn't like. But it took me a while to realize this. For, like a lot of people, I grew up with the mushy Brussels sprouts, canned spinach, revolting beetroot salads and other nameless horrors served in school meals. It was only when I began to make vegetable juices, exuberant salads and to cook my own vegetables that I discovered just how delicious they can be in their many incarnations. When vegetables are cooked properly they have a marvellous flavour of their own. There is little more beautiful to serve with a fish, meat or tofu dish than brightly coloured vegetable purées of carrot, beetroot or spinach. Steam them, stir-fry them, bake them, purée them, eat them raw – however you go, vegetables are not only some of the most important foods in relation to health,

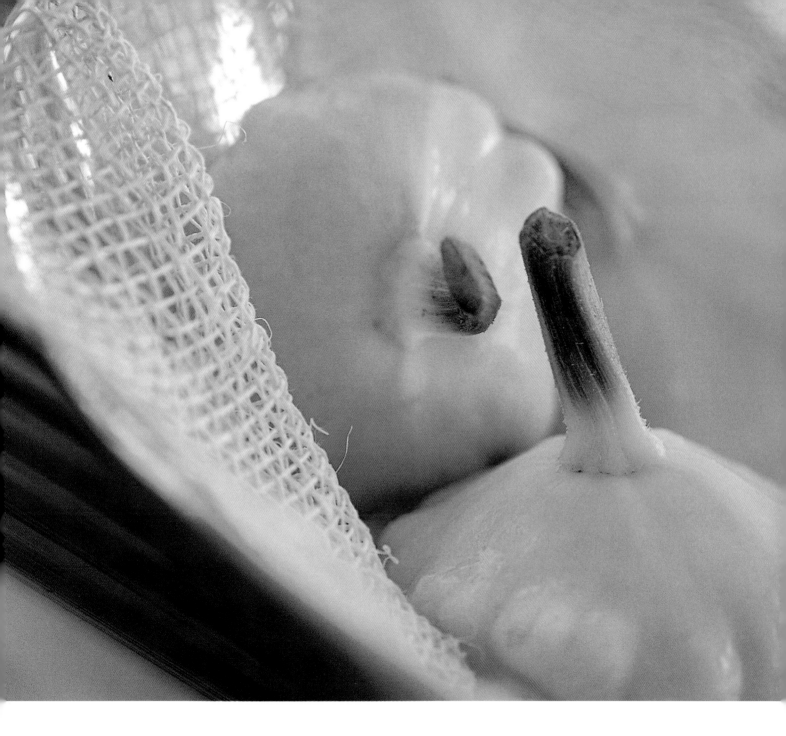

THEY ARE ALSO SOME OF THE

MOST DELICIOUS.

BEYOND ANTIOXIDANTS

Low in both calories and fat and riddled with fibre, fresh vegetables are rich sources of antioxidants from vitamins C and E and the carotenoids to help protect against the free-radical damage which underlies degeneration and early ageing. Not long ago at Tufts University in the United States scientists developed a method of measuring the antioxidant power of specific fruits and vegetables by measuring their ability to quench free radicals in a laboratory test tube. They can now test a food's oxygen radical absorbance capacity. Using the ORAC test, these researchers have begun to categorise a fruit or vegetable according to its overall antioxidant power. They list fruits such as blueberries, strawberries and raspberries at the top along with vegetables like kale, spinach and Brussels sprouts. (For the Inside Story on antioxidants, see page 86.)

Health enhancers

From the humble turnip to the radiant leaves of radicchio, vegetables are also sources of light energy from the sun – the same light energy that 15 billion light years ago created the Universe. Their beauty is the beauty of the life force itself. When they are grown organically in healthy soils and eaten either raw or with as little cooking as possible, this energy, which cannot be measured in chemical terms and whose potential for enhancing health probably goes far beyond even that of the newly discovered phytonutrients, becomes *our* energy.

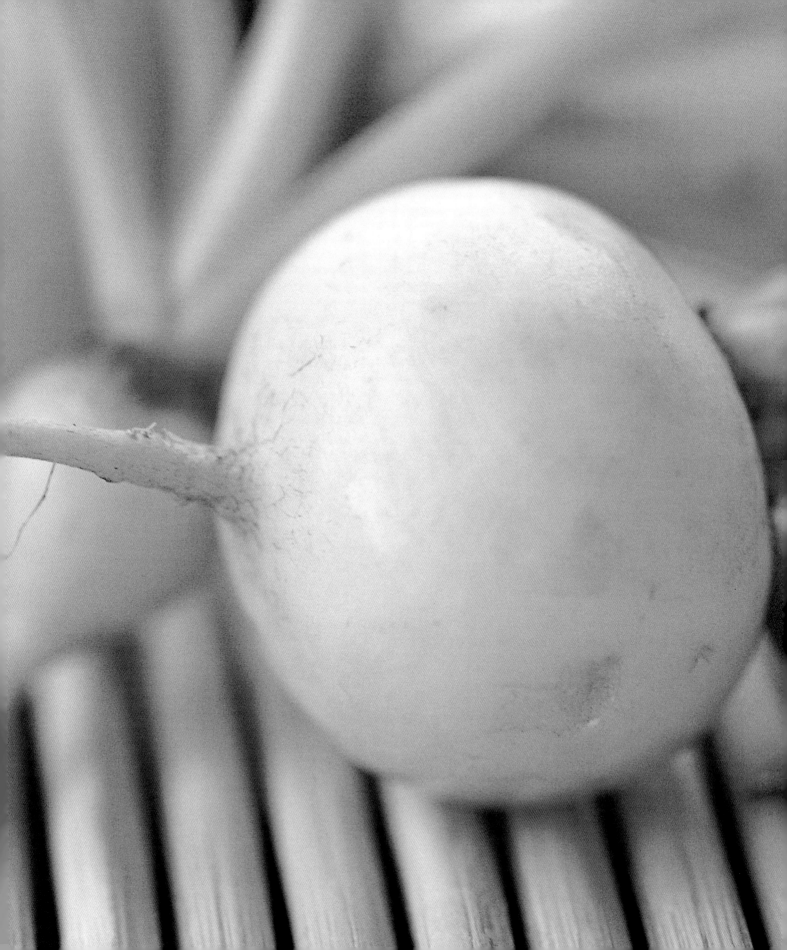

SIGN OF THE CROSS

I always think the word 'cruciferous' sounds like some
kind of a crunchy salad. In fact, it is used to identify
vegetables, such as the brassicas, that get their name
from the fact that they carry cross-shaped flower
petals. These same vegetables – including bok choy,
mustard greens, collards, turnips, swedes, broccoli,
kale, cabbage and cauliflower – boast high levels of all
sorts of phytochemicals and vitamins, plus special kinds
of fibre for long-lasting good looks and high-level well
being. Women who eat a lot of the crucifers – say four
times a week – have a very low incidence of cancer of
the breast and of the ovaries.

Indole-3-carbinol in cruciferous vegetables, and
probably other plant factors too, both help clear the body
of the forms of oestrogen which have a negative effect on
it, as well as help decrease the body's production of
negative oestrogen. To get the best from indoles eat your
vegetables raw, lightly steamed or wok-fried.

Another phytochemical in broccoli – sulphoraphane –
also stimulates the production of anti-cancer and anti-
ageing enzymes in the body. As nature would have it, it
comes packaged up with folic acid, which is a vitamin that
few of us get in adequate quantities. Broccoli has
excellent preventative and protective properties of all
sorts. In terms of both useful fibre and the well-known
antioxidants, vitamins C and A, you would be hard pressed
to get more of these important nutrients from other fruits
and vegetables. Even half a cup of broccoli contains two-
thirds of the recommended daily allowance for vitamin C.
Steam it in a beautiful Chinese steam basket. Then serve it
hot or chill and use in salads.

Green leafy vegetables also contain a phytonutrient
called lutein. A big-league carotenoid antioxidant that
resides in the fatty pigments of plants, lutein keeps
carcinogens from binding to DNA, and in doing so protects
against degenerative diseases including eye diseases. It
also protects cells all over the body, including the skin,
from premature ageing.

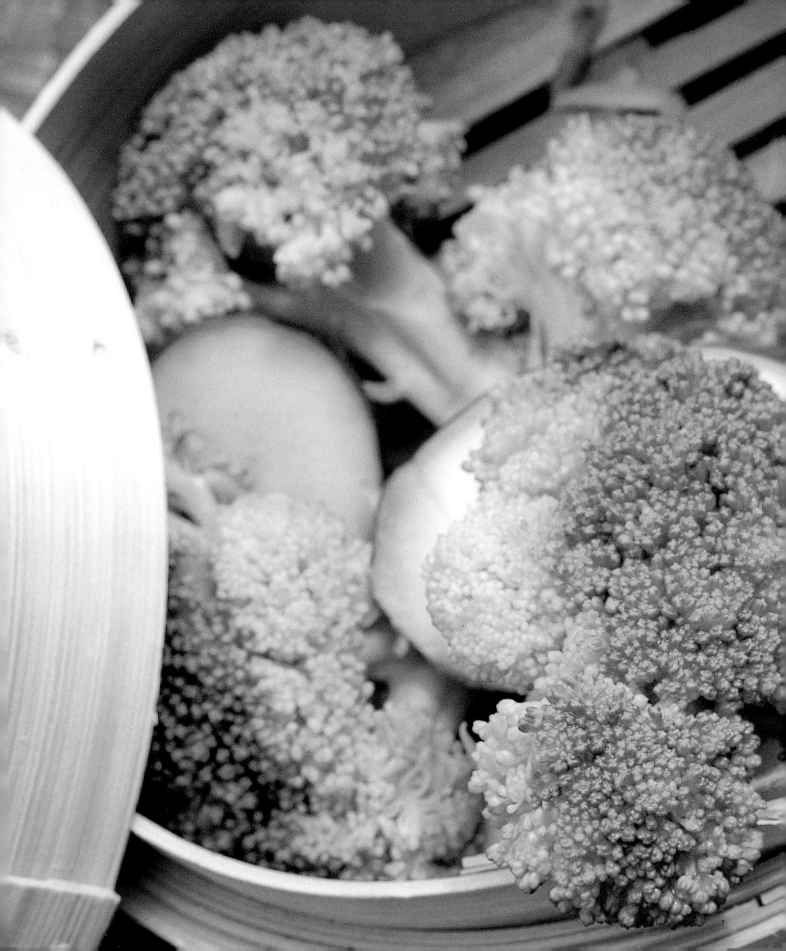

CHAR-GRILLED PEPPERS

serves 4

Another great way of cooking vegetables is to char-grill them with a little olive oil. Peppers make a good vegetable accompaniment to a main course or, as I like to do, you can eat them as a meal on their own, hot or cold, some afternoon or evening when you're not terribly hungry, but want to nibble on something delicious. Many vegetables lend themselves to char grilling. Although this recipe is for peppers, you can carry out the same procedure with red onions, tomatoes, courgettes, aubergines, fennel, celery, cauliflower and broccoli. Even Brussels sprouts, which are by no means my favourite vegetable, come out well when you char grill them. I serve char-grilled vegetables just as they come, marinated in the sauce that I use to baste them while they are under the grill or on the barbecue. Sometimes I squeeze extra lemon over them.

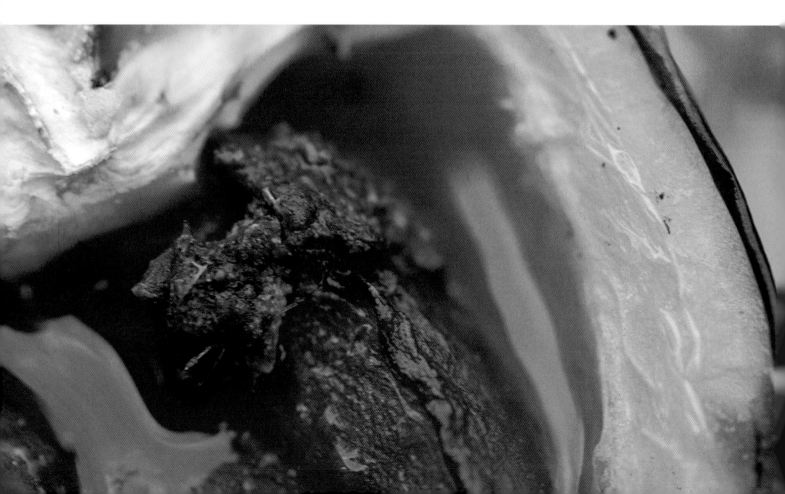

WHAT YOU NEED FOR THE DRESSING

8 tbsp extra-virgin olive oil
1/2 tsp tamari
juice from 1 lime
zest from 1 lime or lemon
1-2 garlic cloves, finely
  chopped
2 tsp red peppercorns, cracked
  with a mortar and pestle
2 tbsp shallots, finely chopped

8 peppers, red, yellow or green
1 red onion, chopped
8 garlic cloves, finely sliced
juice of 1 lemon
small handful of finely chopped
  fresh herbs, e.g. tarragon,
  basil, coriander, flat-
  leaved parsley, fennel, to
  garnish
freshly ground red peppercorns
ribbons of lemon zest

HERE'S HOW

Combine the ingredients of the dressing and mix well. Pour into a flat pan. Cut the peppers in half, remove the seeds and plunge into the dressing. Allow them to sit for between 15 minutes and 3 hours, turning occasionally so that they soak up the dressing. Now you're ready to cook – either on a cast-iron char-grill pan, a teppan yaki grill (**my favourite method, see page 136**), underneath the grill of the oven or atop the barbecue. It is important that the grilling surface is extremely hot.

Place the vegetables backside to the heat first on the grill or pan and cook until brown, turning them over as necessary and brushing on more of the dressing as you go. Turn them and finish off on the open side, filling the centre of the peppers with more of the dressing together with the onions and garlic. Finally, just before serving, squeeze on some lemon and sprinkle with fresh herbs. Alternatively, serve them in a little pile on each dish so that people can sprinkle them over themselves. Add the red peppercorns and serve with ribbons of lemon zest around the vegetables on each plate.

ROAST THEM

Roasting not only helps vegetables maintain their natural flavour, it brings a quality of richness and comfort to any meal. There's something charming about serving a whole baked onion at a meal – amusing as well as delicious. Roasting vegetables is a good method for preserving their vitamins and minerals. Put them in the oven on their own or mix together in a kind of hotpot. If you are lucky enough to have a wood-burning oven (unfortunately I am not – at least not yet), then you will get a special flavour that can't be had any other way.

The best vegetables to roast are the ones like swedes, parsnips, celeriac, carrots, turnips, peppers, summer marrows and courgettes, plus, of course, the perennial onions and garlic. Slice them, dice them (I like to cut them into 12 mm/1/2 in cubes), quarter them or – if they are small – cook them whole.

WHAT YOU NEED

500 g (1 lb 2 oz) vegetables, sliced, diced, quartered or whole, depending upon size
3 tbsp extra-virgin olive oil
Maldon sea salt and freshly ground pepper
fresh chopped herbs, e.g. chives, parsley, rosemary, thyme, sage

HERE'S HOW

Preheat the oven to 200°C/400°F/Gas Mark 6. Place the vegetables in a roasting pan and pour the olive oil over them, seasoning with salt and pepper and mixing with your fingers. Spread them out so that they are in a single layer in the pan. Put into the oven and cook uncovered, stirring occasionally, until they are just beginning to take on a caramel colour. (But beware here: caramelized vegetables taste sweeter, but they are very easy to burn, and if they get too dark they grow bitter.) Now sprinkle with the fresh herbs and serve immediately.

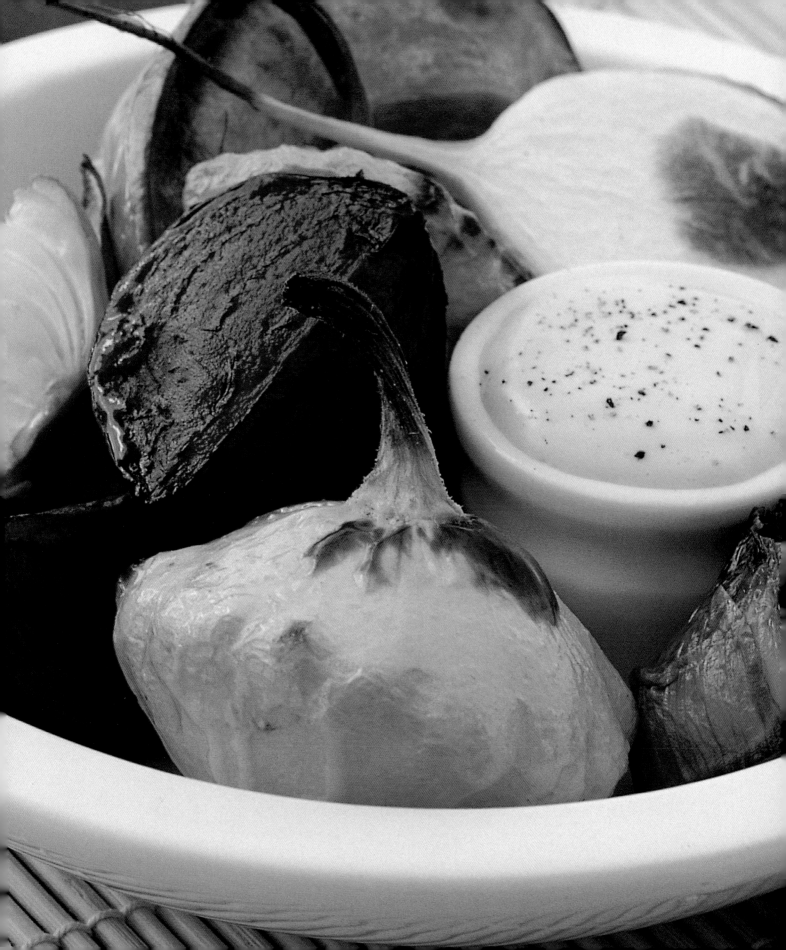

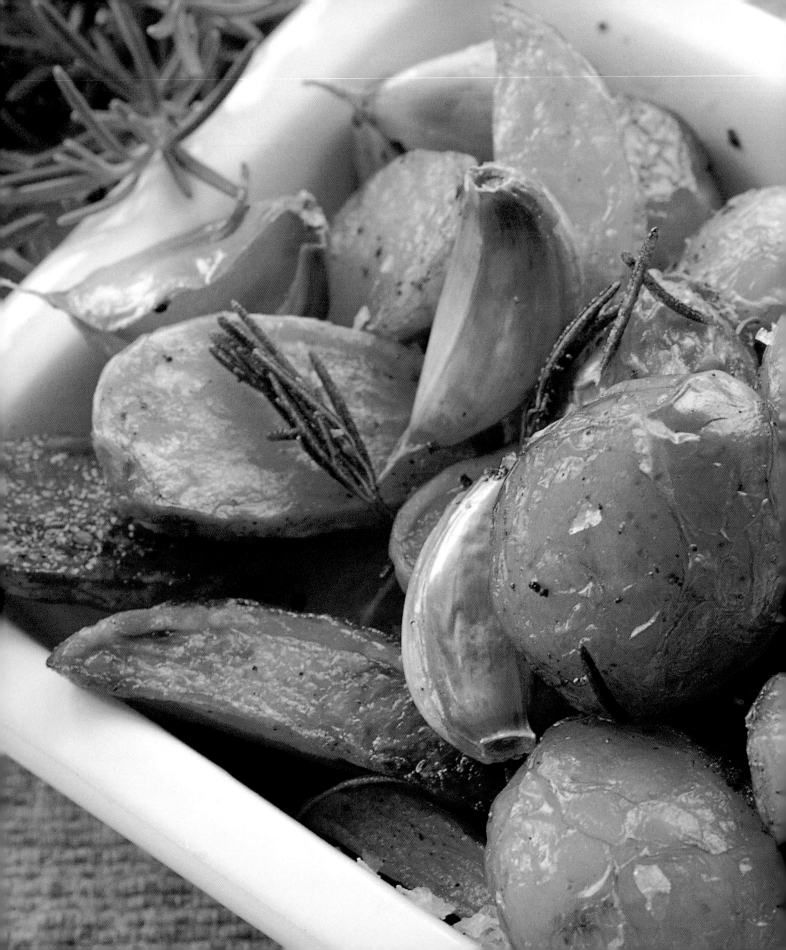

BAKED CHIPS WITH ROSEMARY AND GARLIC

Not only do these chips taste great because they are oven-made, they are not heavy in fat. They contain none of the nasty trans-fatty acids to undermine health that ordinary chips do. You don't even need to peel the potatoes to make them. What you do need to do is ensure the baking sheet is large enough to lay them out flat without overlapping, or they will not cook properly.

I like to make my chips using the thick grating attachment of a mandolin, but you can just as easily cut well-scrubbed potatoes into lengthwise segments. It is useful to have one of those olive oil sprays to use on the baking tin, especially if you want to lower still further the oil content of the chips. I like to use new potatoes or boiling potatoes, but you can also use baking potatoes, especially if you like your chips softer inside.

WHAT YOU NEED
750 g (1 lb 10 oz) potatoes,
   cut into chips
1/4 tsp dried Cajun seasoning
   or 1 tsp fresh (see page 43),
   or more to taste
2 tbsp freshly chopped rosemary
   leaves or 1 1/2 tsp dried
6 garlic cloves, finely chopped
2 or 3 garlic cloves with
   their skin on
Maldon sea salt and freshly
   ground pepper

HERE'S HOW
Preheat the oven to 200°C/400°F/Gas Mark 6. Mix together in a bowl all the ingredients except the potatoes. Now add the potato pieces and toss them with your fingers to coat them well. Put them on to a baking sheet, arranged neatly with spaces to spare. Bake in the oven for 45 minutes, turning them over two or three times until they are lightly browned and tender. Remove the cloves of garlic that are in their skins and use those to decorate the dish. Serve immediately.

BAKED ASPARAGUS

serves 4-6

Not only does asparagus appear in early spring with a very short growing season - which makes it seem ultra-desirable - it is also a powerfully healing vegetable. When shopping for asparagus, look for bright green, straight, fresh-looking spears with compact tips. Stay away from the woody, stringy or streaked spears and those with spreading tips. These are sure signs that they are not really fresh. Bring the asparagus home and rinse it in cold water. Then trim off the bottoms or woody portions. If you have large spears that look tough, peel the outside before cooking.

Because the tips of asparagus cook much faster than the tails, it is a good idea to steam it in a tall, lidded pan designed especially for that purpose. But don't worry if you don't happen to have one; you can also cut it into pieces and pop them into the steamer - the heavier ends first and the little tips afterwards. I like to serve steamed asparagus with wedges of lemon and shaved Parmesan, plus a little garlic salt and pepper. You can also use any of the dips, pestos or mayonnaise including aïoli found in this book and serve asparagus hot or cold. I'm also fond of baked asparagus, cooked as described below. I like to eat it on its own as a meal in itself. (For the Inside Story on asparagus, see page 87.)

WHAT YOU NEED

36 asparagus spears, trimmed and peeled if necessary (see above)
2-6 tbsp melted butter
Maldon sea salt and freshly ground pepper
1 lemon, cut into 6 wedges

HERE'S HOW

Preheat the oven to 220°C/ 425°F/Gas Mark 7. Place the asparagus in a flat baking dish and drizzle with butter. Season with salt and pepper. Cover with a lid or with foil. Then bake in the oven until the spears are browned and tender: 20 to 30 minutes, depending upon the thickness of the asparagus. Add a little extra melted butter just before serving and a wedge of lemon to each plate.

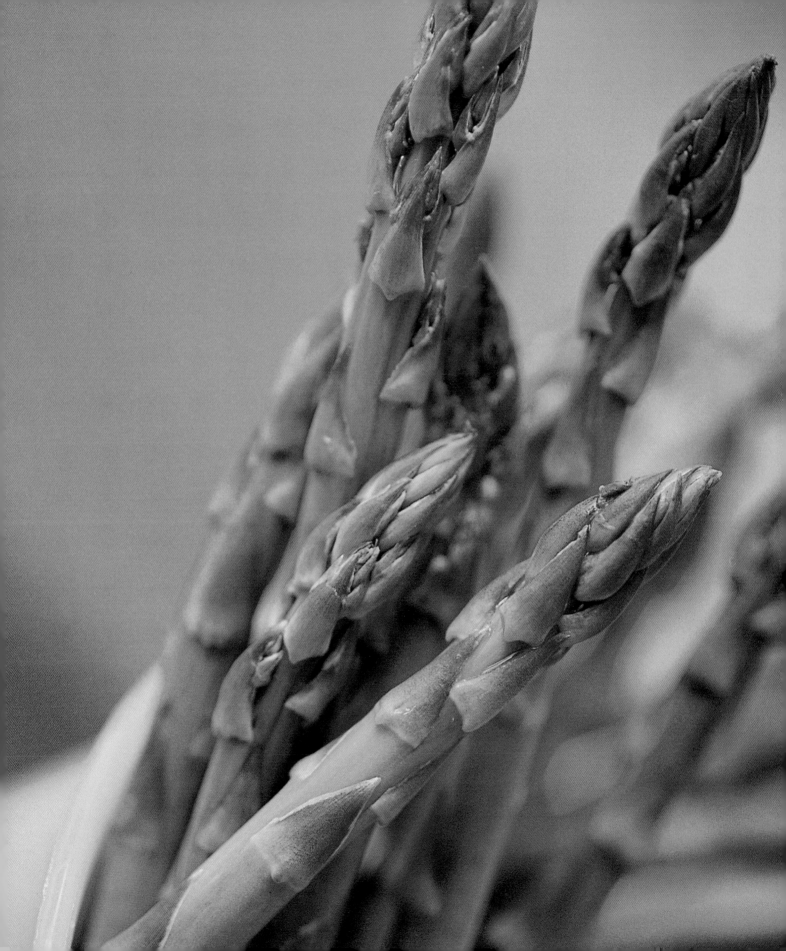

MIDNIGHT FEASTS

10

Around midnight food choices get highly personal. Among the possibilities are foods which induce sleep: raid the refrigerator for turkey sandwich on rye, peel a banana or dip into a bowl of rice pudding. These foods trigger the release of serotonin in the brain, paving the way for blissful sleep.

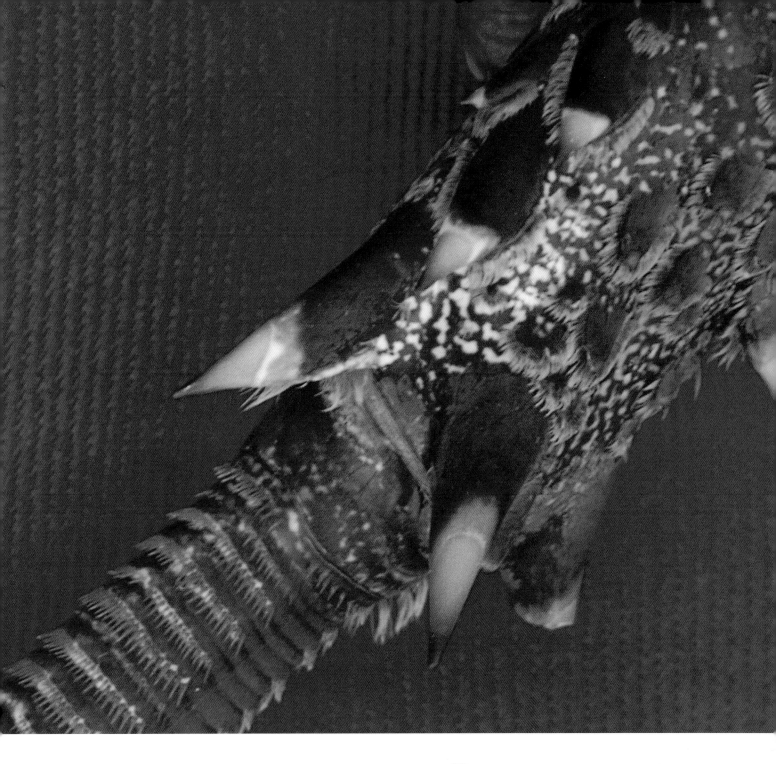

LET INSTINCT BE YOUR GUIDE.

FINE FOODS

LOBSTER OR CRAYFISH WITH DIPPING SAUCES

serves 4

Not only are lobster and crayfish some of the most beautiful foods in nature, they are also some of the most nutritious - especially when it comes to supporting immune functions and reproductive health. Rich in iodine for the thyroid gland and in turn the sex glands, these crustaceans are excellent sources of zinc in a form that your body fairly laps up, of selenium - an essential antioxidant - and of the omega-3 fatty acids, which are strongly linked with their heart-protective and anti-inflammatory properties. Serve with green goddess, blood of angels or midnight sun sauces **(see pages 181-182)**.

WHAT YOU NEED
4 lobsters or crayfish, 400-500 g (14-18 oz) apiece

HERE'S HOW
Once you have chosen your crayfish or lobsters, take them home and put them under a wet towel so they go to sleep. When you are ready to cook them, take a very sharp, thin knife and pith them by sticking the back of the knife through the centre of the neck. It only takes an instant to do. This severs the spinal cord so that when you put them into boiling water they do not suffer. Fill a big pot with enough water to cover and then some. Bring to a rolling boil. Now drop the crayfish or lobsters into the water and cover.

Cook for 3 to 6 minutes, depending on their size. Take them from the pot and put on a board. Now, with a good sharp knife placed just behind the eyes, split them down the top end and then turn around and split the other end so that you are cutting along the entire length. Remove the dark vein that runs down the tail, the stomach sack, which is inside the head, and the gills. Crack open the claws with the base of a large knife. Serve flesh side up with an aïoli **(see page 178)** or dipping sauces **(see page 141)**.

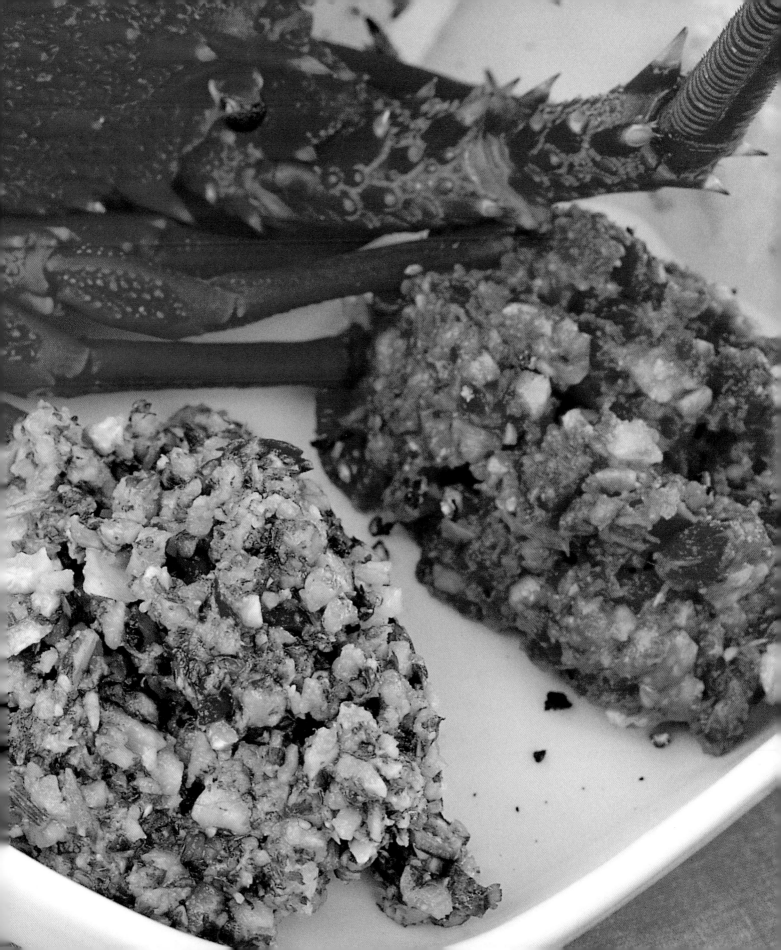

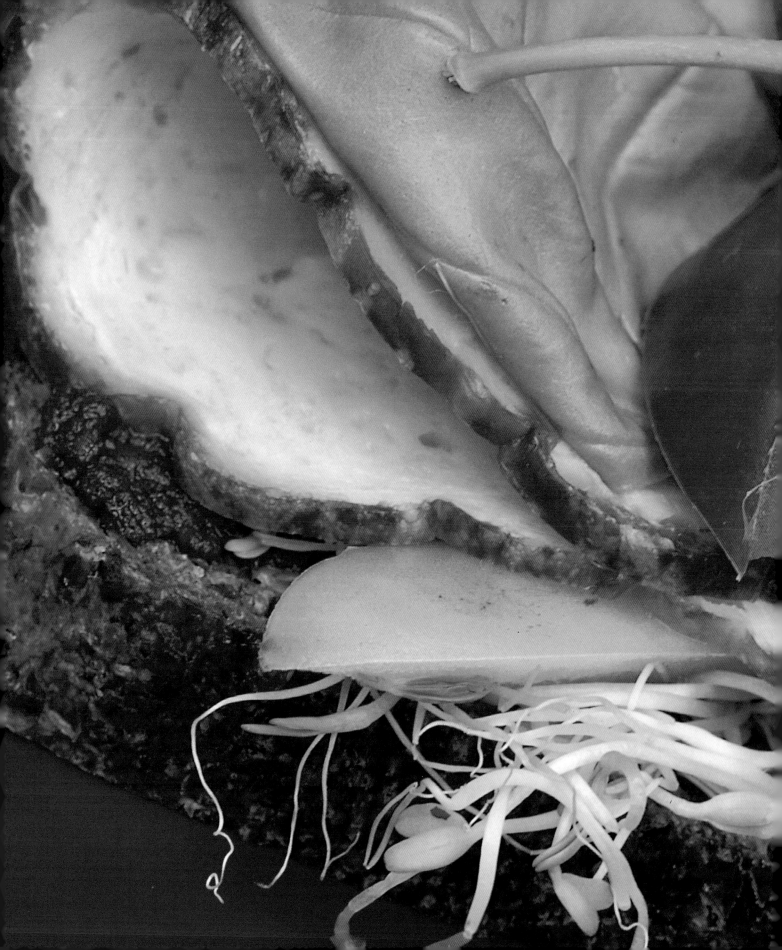

TURKEY SANDWICH ON RYE

Make yourself a turkey sandwich piled high with fresh herbs and sprouts, spread with mayonnaise and topped off with some capers. Why do this just before bed? Because turkey, like bananas, is rich in the amino acid L-tryptophan - which is a natural sedative. In addition to too much wine and fat, this is one reason why after Christmas dinner we can get so sleepy. This amino acid is the starting point from which your body makes serotonin - a brain hormone which calms, reduces appetite and enhances a feeling of well being. Supplements of L-tryptophan were widely used to treat PMS and depression until 1990, when the US Food and Drug Administration banned its sale.

You can make use of L-tryptophan's sedative effect by tucking into a home-made turkey sandwich. Even the rye bread helps further the relaxation process. Grains also encourage the release of serotonin in the brain. Research carried out in the United States showed that eating grains can be a useful practice for those who find themselves becoming stressed day to day. They appear to induce just the right amount of relaxation. However, many women, scientists found, reacted more strongly to eating grains - so strongly in fact that a few became semi-comatose from eating them. Make use of this characteristic of foods when you most want it - just before climbing into bed - to ensure a blissful night's sleep.

BROWN RICE PUDDING

It has to be one of the oldest and most comforting foods in the Western world. Eating rice pudding also brings a soporific state in its wake. You can prepare it way ahead then keep it in the refrigerator for late night raids. Coconut gives this old favourite a new twist.

WHAT YOU NEED
75 g (3 oz) brown rice
900 ml (32 fl oz) coconut
    cream
6 tbsp honey
pinch of salt
pinch of nutmeg
3 tbsp grated almonds
crystallized rose petals or
    toasted slivered almonds,
    to garnish (optional)

HERE'S HOW
Preheat the oven to 130°C/ 250°F/Gas Mark 1/2. Stir all the ingredients together in a casserole dish, except for the rose petals or slivered almonds, and bake uncovered for 3 hours, stirring a couple of times during the first 2 hours. Either serve immediately garnished with crystallized rose petals or slivered almonds or refrigerate for future raids.

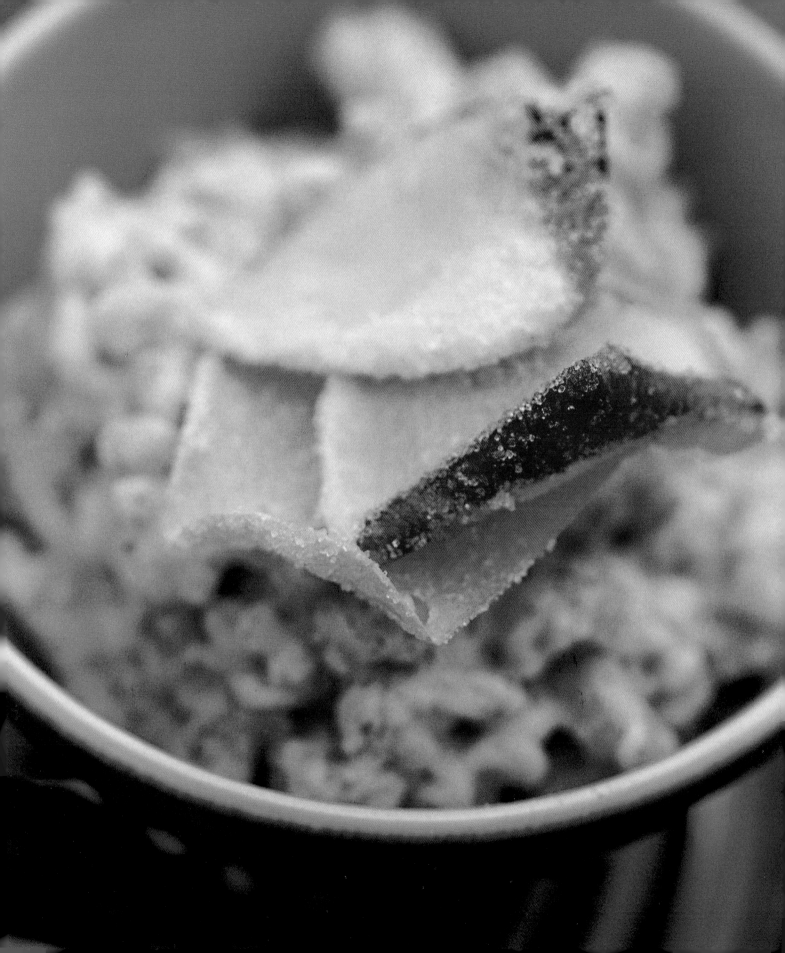

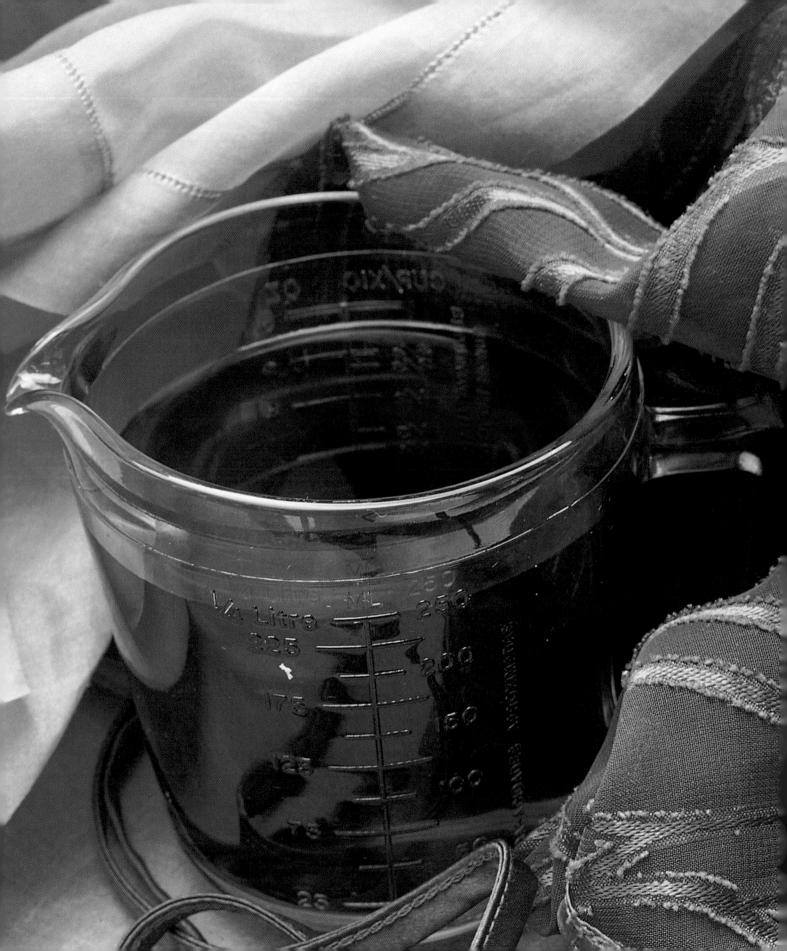

LAVENDER TEA

I know of no more beautiful tea to take at bedtime than this dark midnight brew of tiny fresh lavender flowers. It is relaxing, light and gentle. To brew you need a cafetière and a handful of the flowers. Place them in the cafetière, pour boiling water over them and let steep for between 5 and 15 minutes, depending on how strong you want it. The longer it brews the deeper the violet colour. Press down with the plunger and pour into a glass mug. Serve with a teaspoon of liquid honey just before bed.

THE FRENCH PARADOX

Ten years ago red wine made headlines. Research showed that in spite of the fact that the French eat great volumes of cheese and animal fats - four times as much butter for instance as Americans - the death rate from heart disease is two and a half times lower in France than in the United States. Why? Scientists concluded that it was the amount of red wine the French drink. Immediately, Chardonnay was replaced by Cabernet and Merlot and the sale of Burgundy hit an all time high.

Hearty protection

No more than two glasses of alcohol a day helps protect from heart disease. Red wine is rich in phenolic compounds, which have strong anti-oxidant characteristics. There is strong evidence that when ingested regularly, red wine may contribute to the amelioration of arteriosclerosis and help prevent death by heart disease. Many studies indicate that light drinkers of red wine have less risk of heart problems and death from heart disease than teetotallers. The phenolic compounds, at least in part responsible for protection, include catechins, anthocyanins and tannins, which help prevent the oxidation of LDL cholesterol, inhibiting the likelihood of arteriosclerosis.

serves 4-6

HOLY WINE

Monks have always known the secrets of using alcohol for medicinal as well as aesthetic purposes. In fact, many of the best wines as well as the best liquors were made in monasteries. To me there is little as delicious as a well-made mulled wine as you lie in bed with a lover or sit before the fire with friends talking late into the night. The secret of making the very best is don't skimp on the quality of the wine. Go for a Cabernet Merlot - smooth and mellow - and make sure the spices are fresh. If you wish, you can make this recipe non-alcoholic by substituting a rich red grape juice for the wine. In this case, I add some more lemon zest to the lot. Either way, never use too many different spices or you can confuse the issue and end up with a hotchpotch instead of a blood red miracle of nature.

WHAT YOU NEED

12 cloves
1 organic orange
4 tbsp golden granulated sugar
    or date sugar
4 cinnamon sticks
1 fresh nutmeg, finely grated
zest of 1 lemon, coarsely
    shredded
2 lemons, sliced
750 ml (25 fl oz) dry red wine

HERE'S HOW

Stick the cloves in the flesh of the whole orange and then put it in a big saucepan. Add sugar, cinnamon, nutmeg and lemon slices and zest, reserving a few pieces of the zest to decorate the glasses. Cook over a low heat, stirring occasionally until all the sugar is dissolved. Bring to the boil, then reduce the heat again and simmer for 15 minutes. Now add the red wine, heat through and serve.

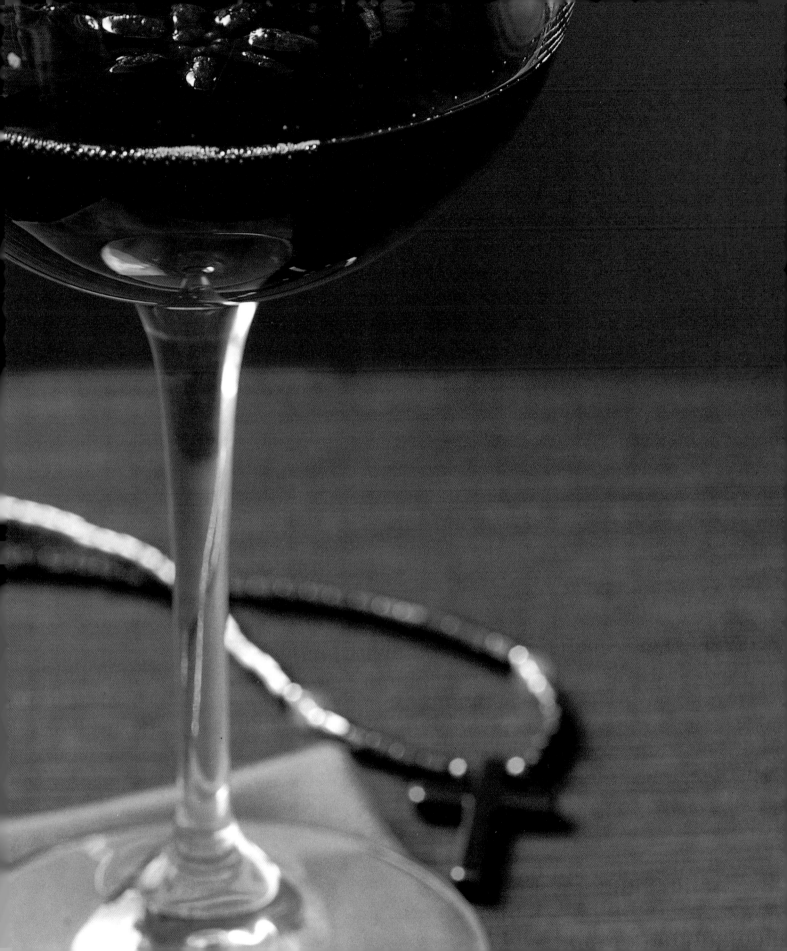

THE BASICS

In addition to all the wonderful, health-enhancing recipes given in this book there are simple ways of making your food taste even better. Here I give you some of my favourite tried-and-tested recipes for stocks, sauces and dips, grains and seeds and low-fat dressings.

HOMEMADE STOCKS

There's an ancient saying that stock to the cook is voice to a singer. I believe it 100 percent. To me stocks make all the difference in the world. I have a passion for not wasting anything, so I like to boil up vegetables, scraps, chicken backs, fish bones — anything that you would ordinarily throw away. I often use lamb bones as well, adding pungent spices to make a meat stock.

FISH STOCK
makes 3 litres (5 1/4 pints)
This stock can be made ahead and kept in the refrigerator for three to four days or in the freezer for three months.

What you need
1 kg (2 lb 4 oz) bones of inexpensive fish that is not too strongly flavoured, e.g. cod, squid, rock cod
3 litres (5 1/4 pints) water
6 stalks of celery
3 fresh bay leaves
bunch of parsley, chopped
2 red onions, roughly chopped
1 fennel bulb or a large bunch of fennel leaves and stalks
3 carrots, sliced
1 garlic head, broken up but unpeeled
300 ml (10 fl oz) white wine
2 sprigs of fresh thyme
Maldon sea salt and freshly ground pepper

Here's how
Toss all the ingredients into a pot and pour boiling water over it and simmer for 20 to 30 minutes. Put through a sieve, throw the bones away and keep the stock. Use immediately, refrigerate immediately or freeze.

CHICKEN STOCK
makes 3 litres (5 1/4 pints)
The whole point of making a stock is to pull out of a carcass or vegetables as much flavour as you possibly can. What you want to do is extract the flavour from the parts of meats and vegetables that we don't usually eat, so it's important to throw every part of the chicken in, as well as any clean vegetable leftovers after making a salad or preparing vegetables for a meal.

What you need
3 chicken carcasses (1.5 kg/3 lb 7 oz) (liver, heart and giblets optional)
3 litres (5 1/4 pints) water
1 leek, sliced
2 onions, chopped
1 lemon, sliced
2 carrots, chopped
1 bunch of parsley
handful of mushrooms, sliced (optional)
4 celery stalks
1 garlic head, broken up but unpeeled
2 sprigs of thyme
3 bay leaves
2 sprigs of fresh rosemary
6 whole black peppercorns

Here's how
In a big pot toss the chicken, water, vegetables, garlic, herbs and seasoning. Bring to the boil then turn down the heat to a simmer and continue to simmer for 3 to 4 hours. Pass the stock through a colander, let it cool for 30 minutes; then put into the refrigerator. After it has cooled, remove the layer of congealed fat from the surface and store or use immediately. I like to divide mine up into convenient-sized refrigerator dishes. You can store this in the refrigerator for four days or in the freezer for two to three months.

VEGETABLE STOCK
makes approximately 3 litres (5 1/4 pints)

What you need
2 large carrots, washed, trimmed and roughly chopped
1/2 garlic head, separated but not skinned
bunch of parsley
1 leek, sliced (optional)
2 onions, chopped
2 bay leaves
1 tsp white peppercorns
1 sprig of rosemary
2 sprigs of thyme
1/2 fennel bulb, chopped (optional)
1/2 celery head, chopped
1 tbsp extra-virgin olive oil
any other vegetables (not asparagus or beetroot) you happen to have in the house, chopped

Here's how
Pop everything into a large stockpot. Add water up to the three-quarter point (about 3 litres/5 1/4 pints). Bring to the boil then reduce the heat and simmer, covered, for 2 hours. Take the cover off the pan and simmer for at least another hour. Strain the stock through a colander and pour into different-sized containers for different uses.

SAUCES AND DIPS

AÏOLI AND AÏOLI LITE
I was introduced to aïoli — an indispensable part of La Bourride (see page 60) — years ago when I lived in Paris. As far as I'm concerned, the taste is overwhelmingly wonderful. I use the very best olive oil I can find when making this rich sauce because I like it strong and true in the Mediterranean way. You can serve this sauce with many things other than fish soup too: hard-boiled eggs, crudités, steamed baby potatoes, fish, sliced cucumbers; you can use it on cold meat, in sandwiches or on freshly baked or steamed fish and on vegetables such as steamed broccoli, mushrooms, beans or spinach. You can also add all sorts of delicious things to aïoli — from toasted slivered almonds to an anchovy or two as well as fresh herbs like basil, lovage or fennel tops — to make many different dips and dressings of it. But I like the simple lemon aïoli best with fish soup.

TRADITIONAL AÏOLI

What you need
1 large egg
1 large egg yolk
juice of 2 ripe lemons
Maldon sea salt and freshly ground pepper
dash of tamari or two pinches of Cajun seasoning (see page 43)
300 ml (10 fl oz) extra-virgin olive oil

2 garlic cloves, finely chopped or crushed
    (less if you are not in love with garlic)
1 tsp Dijon mustard
1-2 tbsp chopped fresh basil, parsley,
    fennel tops or lovage (optional)
1-2 tbsp toasted almond slivers or a
    couple of anchovies (optional)

Here's how
Add the egg, egg yolk and lemon juice
together with the salt and tamari or Cajun
seasoning to a food processor and blend at
high speed. Reduce the speed and slowly –
drop by drop for if you do it faster it will
not emulsify – add the olive oil.

Once you have added about a third of
the olive oil in this way it will have
thickened and then you can add the rest
slowly in a steady stream. Now, turn off
the food processor and either in its own
container or after decanting the mixture to
a bowl, add the garlic, mustard, any herbs
or extras and blend by hand until smooth.
Put in a small crock and serve with your
other dishes or place a spoonful over hot
dishes and watch it melt.

AÏOLI LITE
If you want to steer clear of oil – believe
me traditional aïoli is almost nothing but
oil – why not try my mock aïoli? It too goes
well in fish soups and on any kind of
vegetable.

What you need
450 ml (16 fl oz) soya milk
1 1/2 tbsp arrowroot powder
8 tbsp soya milk powder
1/2 garlic clove, very finely chopped
1 large egg yolk
1-2 tbsp extra-virgin olive oil
lemon juice
1 tsp Dijon mustard
1-2 tbsp chopped fresh basil, dill, fennel
    tops or lovage (optional)
1-2 tbsp toasted almond slivers or a
    couple of anchovies (optional)
freshly ground pepper

Here's how
Place half the soya milk together with the
arrowroot powder in a saucepan. Cook and
stir to thicken. Cool. Into the food
processor put the cooled soya milk and the
soya milk powder and the egg yolk. Blend
well. Slowly add just enough olive oil to
thicken. Add the lemon juice. Remove the

ingredients from the food processor and by
hand mix together the other ingredients.
You can also add some other flavours that
can make it very special, such as chopped
basil, dill, chopped roasted seeds or nuts
and even chopped fennel tops. Season with
black pepper and lemon juice.

LEAN MAYONNAISE
makes about 250 ml (8 fl oz)
This is a spa mayonnaise, very low in fat
but high in protein and taste. It is one of
my favourite recipes – especially good
when you do not want to take in too much
fat in your diet. You can substitute
ordinary mayonnaise for this mayonnaise
in any of the recipes in the book. You can
also mix it with a number of seasonings to
make delicious salad dressings. It will
keep for three to four days in the
refrigerator.

What you need
50 g (2 oz) soft tofu
3 hard-boiled eggs
3 tsp lemon juice
1 tbsp Meaux mustard
2 tbsp finely minced shallots or chives
    (optional)
1/2 tsp organic vegetable bouillon or 1/2
    an organic vegetable bouillon cube
a couple of dashes of Tabasco sauce
    (optional)
a couple of dashes of Worcestershire sauce
    (optional)
Maldon sea salt and freshly ground pepper

Here's how
Put the tofu, egg and lemon juice into a
food processor and purée. Scrape into a
small bowl or jar, then add the remaining
ingredients and let it stand for at least an
hour to absorb the flavour.

ROUILLE
makes about 250 ml (8 fl oz)
I fell in love with rouille when I lived in
Paris – in fact, so in love with it that I
would order bouillabaisse to justify tasting
this chilli-spiked, wild orange mayonnaise.
Once I gathered enough courage and didn't
feel so bad about using it in more
unconventional ways, I began to put it on
steamed vegetables and into soups, and I
even just spread it on toast for open-faced
sandwiches.

My version of rouille is a little bit lower
in olive oil than the classic recipe. For
some of the oil I substitute a couple of
hard-boiled eggs. I know it sounds
unconventional, but it really works a treat.

What you need
1 egg yolk
1 red chilli, de-seeded and finely chopped
2 hard-boiled eggs
3 garlic cloves, finely chopped
4 tbsp extra-virgin olive oil
1 tbsp ground almonds
3-4 sun-dried tomatoes, finely chopped
cayenne pepper
Maldon sea salt
Freshly ground pepper

Here's how
Place the egg yolk and chopped chilli in a
food processor. Pop in the 2 hard-boiled
eggs plus a little bit of water and process
until it becomes a smooth paste. While the
machine is still running, add the oil drop
by drop until you get a creamy, thick
sauce. If it gets too thick, add a little more
water. Add the almonds, sun-dried
tomatoes and season to taste. Chill or
serve immediately. It will keep for two to
three days in the refrigerator.

COCONUT CREAM SAUCE
This is a sauce you can use just about
anywhere and it works beautifully over
steamed cabbage, broccoli, cauliflower,
spinach, fish, chicken or lamb – in fact
over just about anything. You can make it
with fresh coconut liquid, in which case
you need to mix it with a bit of arrowroot in
order to thicken, or you can make it – as I
usually do – with canned coconut milk.

What you need
3 tbsp cold-pressed sesame oil
1 small onion, finely chopped
2 garlic cloves, finely chopped
300 ml (10 fl oz) coconut milk
1/8 tsp Cajun seasoning (see page 43)
1/2 tsp ground turmeric
Maldon sea salt and freshly ground red
    peppercorns
2 tbsp broad-leaved parsley or fresh
    coriander, finely chopped

Here's how
Put the sesame oil into a pan and fry the
onions and garlic until very light brown.

Now add the coconut, Cajun seasoning, turmeric and other seasonings except the chopped herbs. Cook for 2 or 3 minutes until heated through; then remove from heat. Add the fresh herbs, reserving a teaspoonful as a garnish, and pour into a bowl or directly over the vegetables or fish that you're serving the sauce with. Garnish with the rest of the chopped fresh herbs. If you prefer your sauce thicker, thicken with a little arrowroot or cornstarch.

AUBERGINE DIP
serves as many as you like
I make a delicious dip for crudités from aubergines. I bake them whole in the oven until their skin goes black and blistered and their flesh goes soft. It's easy to make, provided you don't forget – as I often do – that you've put the aubergines in the oven. Otherwise you'll end up – as I often have – with black, puffed-up footballs, so over-cooked that there is virtually nothing left inside them.

What you need
2 good-sized aubergines
2 garlic cloves, finely chopped
100 g (4 oz) raw cashew nuts
4 tbsp sesame seeds
juice of 1/2 a lemon
1/2 tsp ground cumin
1-2 tbsp extra-virgin olive oil
pinch of cayenne
Maldon sea salt

Here's how
Preheat the oven to 200ºC /400ºF / Gas Mark 6. Prick the aubergines with a fork to ensure they don't explode and place on a baking tray. Roast them until they are soft and their skin black and blistered. This usually takes about 45 minutes. Cool. Tear off the charred skin and discard. Squeeze out as much water as you can from the flesh, then put the aubergines, garlic and cashews into a food processor and blend until smooth. Add the sesame seeds, lemon juice, cumin and olive oil and blend again till smooth. Season with cayenne and salt to taste. Cover and set aside for 45 minutes to let the flavours blend. Then serve the aubergine mixture chilled as a dip for plenty of fresh crudités, as a topping for steamed vegetables or baked potatoes, or as a delicious spread on crackers or toast.

TAPENADE
makes about 450 ml (16 fl oz)
I love good olives. One of the nicest ways to eat them is to combine them with capers, garlic and fresh herbs to make a tapenade – a paste that you can use as a dipping sauce, to put over vegetables or pasta or simply to spread on toast at tea. This is one of the easiest spreads to make – it takes only about 5 minutes. It is best served chilled.

What you need
1 x 250 g (9 oz) can good quality black olives with pits removed
2 tbsp capers, washed and dried
4 anchovy fillets, chopped
2 tbsp fresh lemon juice
2-3 tbsp extra-virgin olive oil
1 tbsp fresh basil, chopped
1 tsp fresh oregano, finely chopped
1-2 garlic cloves, finely chopped

Here's how
Put all the ingredients except the olive oil, herbs and garlic into a food processor and blend until creamy. Now gently and slowly add the olive oil drop by drop. Should the mixture become too thick, add a little more olive oil until you get the right consistency. Pour into a bowl or jar, add the herbs and garlic and mix with a fork. Cover and chill. This will keep for two to three days in the refrigerator.

CURRIED GUACAMOLE
makes about 600 ml (20 fl oz)
This is my version of guacamole. It relies for its flavour on the usual ingredients – onion, lemon juice, coriander, chopped tomato and peppers – but then calls for a couple of teaspoons of medium curry powder and a teaspoon of the miraculous youth spice turmeric. This sauce or dip – depending on how thick you choose to make it goes beautifully with oven-roasted chips, fresh vegetables and as a dip for any kind of crudités.

I prefer not to make guacamole in a food processor because I actually like the hand-made quality of it – too smooth and it lacks interest. However, if you want a smoother guacamole, you can always put it in the food processor. You might need to use a little bit less tomato, however, or it can become too runny.

What you need
2 ripe avocados
3 tbsp fresh lemon juice
3 tbsp chopped tomatoes
2 tbsp coriander
1-2 tsp mild to medium curry powder
1 tsp turmeric
4 shallots, finely sliced
Maldon sea salt
Cajun seasoning (see page 43) or 1/2 tsp store-bought Cajun seasoning

Here's how
Cut the avocados in half and remove the stones. Scoop them out and place the contents in a bowl. Drizzle with lemon juice and mash. Add the chopped tomatoes, coriander and curry powder and turmeric, as well as the rest of the lemon juice and sliced shallots and mix well. Season to taste.

SUN-DRIED TOMATO PESTO
serves as many as you like
There is something magic about the taste of sun-dried tomatoes. I know no better way to honour their earthy beauty than to make a pesto from them. This one is delicious as a dip for crudités. It also makes a wonderful spread on home-baked crackers or bread. The traditional way of eating pesto, of course, is on focaccia bread and certainly it is delicious this way. However, I like it even better on a good, rich, sourdough rye. When choosing the sun-dried tomatoes, you want simple dried tomatoes themselves, not the kind you can buy packed in oil.

What you need
24 sun-dried tomatoes
75 g (3 oz) unsalted macadamia nuts
150 g (5 oz) fresh basil leaves removed from the stem
3 garlic cloves
1 1/2 tbsp tomato paste
1 1/2 tbsp balsamic vinegar
3 tsp lemon juice
250 ml (8 fl oz) tomato juice
4 tbsp extra-virgin olive oil
Maldon sea salt and freshly ground pepper

Here's how
If the sun-dried tomatoes are not soaked in oil in a jar, put them in a small bowl and cover with 450 ml (16 fl oz) of boiling water. Soak them until they go soft – this

usually takes about 20 minutes. Pop them into a food processor with the macadamias, basil, garlic, tomato paste, vinegar, lemon juice, tomato juice and the olive oil and purée, being sure to scrape down the sides several times until the pesto is smooth. Remove from the food processor into a bowl, season – be sure to season generously if you're going to use the pesto on pasta or as a sauce for a baked potato. Use the pesto right away, or it will store for up to five days in a refrigerator.

This also makes a terrific salad dressing if you use a little bit more tomato juice to make it thinner. Use immediately or, poured into small jars or plastic containers, this pesto will keep in the refrigerator for a week, especially if you brush the surface of the pesto with a little olive oil before closing the jar. Pesto does freeze, but you lose some of the flavour. I sometimes fill ice trays with pesto and then remove the cubes and store them in sealed bags, taking out one or two at a time as I need them. They need to thaw at room temperature before being used on top of a vegetable dish or some other dish.

BASIL PESTO
makes a medium-sized bowlful
Basil is my favourite herb. I'm sure I use it in excess just because I so adore how it smells and tastes. (For the Inside Story on basil, see page 90.)

What you need
50 g (2 oz) fresh basil leaves
3 tbsp pine nuts
4 tbsp extra-virgin olive oil
a little lemon juice
25 g (1 oz) fresh Parmesan cheese, finely grated
2 garlic cloves, finely chopped

Here's how
Pop all of the ingredients except the garlic and the Parmesan cheese into a food processor and blend to break them up (but not so much that you turn them into a purée). Keep stopping and scraping things down from the sides of the processor and blend again. If you need extra moisture add a teaspoon or more of fresh lemon juice. Once the sauce takes on a creamy texture (yet, hopefully, still maintains the pieces of basil so that you can see them)

add the Parmesan cheese and the garlic and quickly blend again, then chill.

Serve on dark bread, as a dip or spread on crackers. You can also put it over cooked vegetables and omelettes. Store the sauce in the refrigerator for two days or serve as soon as it is cool. You can also dilute it whenever you wish, by adding a little more lemon juice.

CORIANDER SALSA
makes a medium-sized bowlful
This salsa is made with fresh coriander – lots of it – and cashews and is particularly good served with lamb or chicken. Cashews have the ability to bind almost any foods that you mix them with to create a creamy, sensuous food experience. This is a salsa I created one day when I had virtually nothing in the house but a bag full of nuts, but the garden was brimming with fresh herbs. I think you'll like its unusual flavour and texture.

What you need
200 g (7 oz) fresh raw cashews
3 bunches of coriander (both leaves and stems)
2 medium-hot red chillies, de-seeded and chopped
finely shredded zest of 2 limes
juice of 2 limes
3 tbsp extra-virgin olive oil
1-3 garlic cloves, chopped (optional)
Maldon sea salt and freshly ground pepper

Here's how
Place all the ingredients in a food processor and blend until the mixture is just combined. Chill and serve.

TOFU DIP
serves as many as you like
This is what I call a dip-dressing. It's a thick dressing that you can use as a dip for crudités, or you can thin it with a little spring water and use it to dress a salad.

What you need
250 g (9 oz) tofu
1 tsp wholegrain Meaux mustard
1 tsp organic vegetable bouillon powder or 1/2 an organic bouillon cube
a few leaves of fresh basil and mint
juice and zest of 1 lemon, finely shredded
extra basil leaves

HERE'S HOW
Place all the ingredients except the lemon zest and extra basil leaves into a food processor and blend until creamy. Remove. Add the lemon zest and a few extra chopped leaves of basil.

GREEN GODDESS SAUCE
Makes a medium-sized bowlful

What you need
1 ripe avocado
handful watercress leaves, finely chopped
2 tbsp spring onions
juice of 1 lime
1/2 tsp vegetable bouillon powder
1 garlic clove

Here's how
Place the ingredients in a food processor and pulse on and off to blend, being careful not to blend too much so that the texture of the chopped vegetables remains intact.

BLOOD OF ANGELS SAUCE
Makes a medium-sized bowlful

What you need
2 small tomatoes
small handful of sun-dried tomatoes
small handful of cashews
1 tsp fresh thyme or oregano, finely chopped
a dash or two of Worcestershire sauce
juice of 1 lemon
1 tsp finely grated ginger

Here's how
Place the tomatoes, sun-dried tomatoes, cashews, thyme or oregano, Worcestershire sauce and lemon juice in a food processor and blend until smooth. Now add the grated ginger and stir in by hand. Put in the refrigerator to chill so the flavours blend.

MIDNIGHT SUN SAUCE
Makes a medium-sized bowlful

What you need
2 yellow peppers
1 shallot
1 garlic clove
250 ml (8 fl oz) mayonnaise or soya
    mayonnaise
1 feather of saffron
1/2 tsp turmeric
juice of 1 lemon

Here's how
Blend all ingredients together in a food
processor and serve.

LIGHT WHIPPED TOPPING
Makes 500 ml (16 fl oz)
There are a number of delicious light
toppings you can make to go on sweets,
fruits, jellies and even as dips for fruit
crudités. Here's the standard one that I
use. It's made from soya milk and cold-
pressed sesame oil. There are many
different things you can add to it to give it
a special flavour and colour, depending on
what you want to serve it with.

What you need
250 ml (8 fl oz) soya milk
250 ml (8 fl oz) cold-pressed sesame oil or
    Udo's Choice (see Resources)
1/2 tsp vanilla extract
2-3 tbsp honey
pinch of salt

Here's how
Put the milk into a food processor and turn
on at high speed. Very slowly add the oil —
almost as though you are making
mayonnaise. It will gradually thicken. Keep
your eye on it, as you may need to add a
little extra oil. Finally blend in the vanilla
extract, honey and salt.

GRAINS AND SEEDS
Here are some of my favourite grain
dishes. They can themselves be the basis
of a main meal served together with a
salad or vegetables. Grains are particularly
good for athletes since they are the
lightest form of complex carbohydrates to
release energy slowly over many hours
while you work or exercise. Each grain has
its own natural characteristic. The

important thing is to vary the grains that
you eat, for each grain also has its own
synergistic complements of vitamins and
minerals. Grains are a greatly satisfying
food that, because of their action on the
brain chemical serotonin, help keep you
calm and feeling emotionally supported.

YUMMY BROWN RICE
serves 4
Rice cooked in this manner is so delicious
that it seems to be a worthwhile dish in
itself. It needs no special sauces or
condiments to make it work.

What you need
175 g (6 oz) brown rice
450-720 ml (16-25 fl oz) water
2 tsp vegetable bouillon powder
1 tsp marjoram
2 garlic cloves, finely chopped (optional)
3 tbsp fresh parsley, chopped

Here's how
Wash the rice three times under running
water and put into a saucepan. Boil the
water in a kettle and pour over the rice.
Add the vegetable bouillon powder,
marjoram and garlic. Bring to the boil and
cook gently, covered, for 45 minutes or
until all the liquid has been absorbed.
Garnish with parsley and serve. If you
double the quantities used here you can
keep some back and make a delicious rice
salad the next day.

KASHA
serves 4-6
Kasha has been a favourite for me ever
since a Russian lover taught me how to
make this traditional dish. It makes a
wonderful breakfast — especially to share
in bed on a Sunday morning.

What you need
250 g (8 oz) buckwheat
1 litre (1 3/4 pints) spring water
2 tsp low-salt vegetable bouillon powder or
    1 litre (1 3/4 pints) stock (see page
    178)
2 tbsp chopped fresh parsley or other
    herbs
1 garlic clove, crushed

Here's how
Place the buckwheat in a heavy-bottomed

pan and roast it dry over a medium heat
while stirring with a wooden spoon. As it
begins to darken pour hot water over it and
add the vegetable bouillon powder (if
using water rather than stock), garlic and
1 teaspoon of the herbs. Cover and simmer
very slowly for about 15 to 20 minutes
until all the liquid has been absorbed.
Serve sprinkled with the remaining herbs
or pour a light gravy over the top.

POLENTA
serves 4
Polenta is a peasant dish made from
cornmeal. I particularly like it served with
a salad dressed with a spicy sauce.

What you need
720 ml (1 1/4 pints) spring water
2 tsp low-salt vegetable bouillon powder or
    720 ml (1 1/4 pints) stock (see page
    178)
100 g (4 oz) cornmeal

Here's how
Heat the water or stock. Pour it over the
cornmeal and blend into a paste with the
vegetable bouillon powder (if using water
rather than stock). Stir until smooth and
cook very gently until all the liquid has
been absorbed. Cool and drop by the
spoonful on to a very lightly oiled baking
sheet and grill until brown, turning once.

MILLET
serves 4
Once used by the Romans to make
porridge, millet is still an important staple
in many parts of Africa. It is a bland and
highly nutritious grain that contains all of
the essential amino acids plus an excellent
complement of the B-complex vitamins
and minerals.

What you need
1 litre (1 3/4 pints) spring water
2 tsp low-salt vegetable bouillon powder or
    1 litre (1 3/4 pints) stock (see page
    178)
175 g (6 oz) millet
1 medium onion, finely chopped
1 tsp paprika
2 tbsp chopped parsley

Here's how
Boil the stock or water and pour it over the

millet in a deep saucepan. Add the vegetable bouillon powder (if using water rather than stock), onion, paprika and half of the parsley. Cook over low heat for 30 to 45 minutes until all the liquid has been absorbed. Sprinkle with the remainder of the parsley and serve.

Cooked millet can be formed into small balls together with grated carrots, finely chopped onions, a little parsley and a little lemon juice and served cold as part of a salad.

BARLEY PILAFF
serves 4
A delicious baked dish, barley pilaff is made from pot barley rather than from pearl barley (too many of the B-complex vitamins and minerals have been removed from pearl barley). Barley is also excellent used in soups.

What you need
2 onions, finely chopped
1 tsp extra-virgin olive oil
100 g (4 oz) pot barley
500 ml (16 fl oz) spring water
1 tbsp low-salt vegetable bouillon powder or 250 ml (8 fl oz) stock (see page 178)
1 tbsp dill
2 garlic cloves, finely chopped (optional)

Here's how
Sauté the onions in the oil until translucent, then add the barley to the saucepan and stir well. Remove from the heat and add the remaining ingredients. Place in a lightly oiled oven dish and bake, covered, in a moderate oven for 30 minutes. Check to see if you need to add a little more water. Serve immediately.

THREE TOASTED SEED TOPPINGS
makes 200 g (7 oz)
One of the most delicious things you can do to contrast the light crunchiness of a fresh salad is to top it off with spiced, toasted seeds. The toasting brings out the flavour of seeds or nuts because it helps release the essential oils. You can add them to soups and cooked vegetable dishes. When you are buying any kind of seeds make sure that they are truly fresh. Far too often they sit on shelves in stores too long and lose their healthy properties. Like nuts, ideally they should be stored in

a refrigerator. (For the Inside Story on seed power, see page 88.)

What you need
175 g (6 oz) sesame, pumpkin and/or sunflower seeds
3 tbsp organic bouillon powder or 1 1/2 organic vegetable bouillon cubes, crumbled
1 garlic clove, very finely chopped
1 tbsp onion flakes (optional)

Here's how
Heat a large, heavy, dry pan on the stove and lightly toast the seeds until they go a beautiful brown. Be careful not to overcook them, or you can toast them in the oven for 15 minutes at 150°C /300°F/Gas Mark 2. Be sure to stir them frequently. Then add the other ingredients while still warm and blend well. Sprinkle them liberally over warm vegetables or fresh salads.

SPROUT IT YOURSELF
For small quantities, grow your seeds in glass jars covered with nylon mesh held in place with an elastic band around the neck. For larger amounts, grow them on paper kitchen towels in seed trays with drainage holes that are available from gardening shops and nurseries.

What you need
seeds or beans
jar or bowl to soak seeds
nylon sieve
cheesecloth or stainless-steel sprouting screen or seed trays
kitchen paper towels
plant atomizer
nylon sieve

Here's how
Place two handfuls of seeds or beans in the bottom of a jar or bowl and cover with plenty of water — use at least one part seed to three parts water. Leave to soak overnight. Pour the seeds into a sieve and rinse well with water. Be sure to remove any dead or broken seeds or pieces of debris. If you are using glass jars then return the soaked seeds to the jar after rinsing well and cover with the cheesecloth or sprouting screen secured with a rubber band, drain well and keep in a warm dark place. They can even be covered with a bag or a cloth to create the darkness.

Rinse thoroughly twice a day and be sure to drain them well or you will find they may draw mould.

If you are using a tray, line it with moist kitchen paper towels and pour in the soaked seeds. Place in a warm, dark spot for fast growth. Spray the seeds twice a day with fresh water in the atomizer and stir them gently with your hand to aerate them.

Some sprouts, such as radish or mustard for instance, are zesty and add fire to any dish. They mix well with milder sprouts such as alfalfa or mung. While they are sprouting, the hulls of some seeds come off — usually while you are rinsing them. Discard the hulls as they tend to rot easily. You can do this by placing the sprouts in a big bowl of water and shaking it gently to separate the hulls from the sprouts themselves. Usually the hulls sink to the bottom.

After about three days, place the seeds in sunlight for several hours to develop the chlorophyll in them. Rinse in a sieve, drain well and put in a polythene bag in the refrigerator to use in salads, stir-fries, etc. There are many different seeds you can sprout, each with its own particular flavour and texture.

LOW-FAT DRESSINGS
Whoever said that low-fat dressings have no flavour? Not when they are skilfully blended for texture and spiked with garlic or fresh herbs. Some of these might surprise you. Don't be afraid to experiment with them. You can make some of them out of surprising leftovers —brown rice from the night before, or lentils or chick peas. Any of these can make a great base for a creamy dressing. Most of the dressings here call for simple ingredients and supermarket spices such as garlic salt, onion powder or Cajun seasoning — unless you wish to make your Cajun seasoning as given on page 43. Be sure to season each to taste and don't be afraid to add an extra ingredient or two whenever you feel the dressing needs it. The more inventive you become the better they get.

DRESSING THE SALAD
I tend to be lazy about salad dressings. Often as not, I make my salad in a large flat bowl and then, instead of mixing the

salad dressing separately, I will dress the salad right there and then: a few tablespoons of extra-virgin olive oil, some chopped fresh herbs, a dash of Worcestershire sauce, some Maldon sea salt, the juice of a lemon or a couple of tablespoons of balsamic vinegar, some home-made Cajun seasoning from the refrigerator (or a dash of the powdered variety from the market). To top it off, I add some freshly ground coarse black pepper, ground with a mortar and pestle because it tastes so much better that way. I sprinkle it all on top and toss. Salad: ready in an instant. Sometimes I'll top off my salads with seeds like pumpkin, sesame or sunflower. Others I scatter with fresh garlic or wild garlic leaves, when they are growing down the path near where I live. I add some fresh edible flowers like marigold petals or heartsease. In this section you will find lots of suggestions for salad dressings and toppings.

SUNNY TOMATO DRESSING
makes a medium-sized bowlful
A surprising combination of the tangy flavour of tomatoes sprinkled with herbs.

What you need
6 tomatoes
175 g (6 oz) cooked lima beans, chick peas, brown rice or even leftover potatoes
2 tsp organic vegetable bouillon powder
1 garlic clove, finely chopped
juice of 2 lemons
1 tbsp fresh parsley or fresh basil, finely chopped
dash of Worcestershire sauce
pinch of Cajun seasoning (see page 43)

Here's how
Put the ingredients in a food processor and blend thoroughly. The dressing will thicken as it stands. Thin with spring water if you want a thinner consistency. Chill thoroughly before use. This dressing will keep for two days in the refrigerator.

SPROUT SALAD DRESSING
makes enough to dress a salad for 4

What you need
50 g (2 oz) tofu or 3 medium ripe tomatoes
100 g (4 oz) fresh garden herbs

1 tbsp sesame seeds
2 tbsp lemon juice
Maldon sea salt and freshly ground pepper
1 tbsp shallots, finely chopped
1 tbsp celery, finely chopped

Here's how
Place all ingredients except the shallots and celery in a food processor and mix well. Then remove from the food processor and blend in the chopped shallots and celery by hand. Can be used as a dip or a dressing.

OLIVE OIL, BASIL AND LEMON DRESSING
makes a large salad

What you need
2 tbsp fresh lemon juice
5 tbsp extra-virgin olive oil
handful of fresh basil leaves
1 tsp Maldon sea salt
zest of 1/2 lemon, shredded fine
freshly ground pepper

Here's how
Place all the ingredients except the lemon zest and pepper into a food processor. Blend until smooth. Add the lemon zest and pepper and pour over the salad.

WHOLEGRAIN MUSTARD AND GARLIC DRESSING
makes a large salad

What you need
5 tbsp extra-virgin olive oil
2 tbsp lemon juice
1 tbsp Meaux mustard
1 tbsp liquid honey (I prefer manuka because of its strong flavour)
3 garlic cloves, finely chopped

Here's how
Mix together all the ingredients and pour over the salad.

LEAN VINAIGRETTE
makes 250 ml (8 fl oz)
This is the leanest vinaigrette I have ever come across – so lean that it comes out at less than 25 calories per tablespoon. It depends for its flavour on fresh herbs – whatever you happen to have on hand:

curry plant, savoury, basil, tarragon, thyme, oregano, lovage (the fresher the better) together with pressed garlic or a dash or two of Cajun seasoning. I like to make it with Udo's Choice (see Resources). But it is equally delicious with cold-pressed walnut oil, or extra-virgin olive oil for that matter. Once you make the dressing it will keep in the refrigerator for a week. In fact, it's a good idea to make it a day or two before you need it, since the flavour of the herbs improves the flavour of the vinaigrette.

What you need
4 tbsp Udo's Choice, cold-pressed walnut oil or extra-virgin olive oil
4 tbsp rice wine vinegar or balsamic vinegar
4 tbsp grape juice or mineral water
3 tbsp fresh lemon juice
finely shredded zest from 1/2 a lemon
2 tbsp Meaux mustard
2 tbsp chopped chives
1 tsp Cajun seasoning (see page 43) or 1/2 tsp shop-bought Cajun seasoning
2 garlic cloves, finely chopped (optional)
3 tbsp fresh herbs of your choice, e.g. curry plant, savoury, basil, tarragon, thyme, oregano, lovage

Here's how
Place all the ingredients together in a jar and shake together to blend. Cover tightly and put into the refrigerator to chill and steep.

TOFU VINAIGRETTE
makes enough to dress a salad for 4

What you need
75 g (3 oz) tofu
3 tbsp wine vinegar
juice of 2 lemons
1 tbsp Dijon mustard
1 garlic clove, crushed
Maldon sea salt and freshly ground pepper

Here's how
Place all the ingredients in a food processor and process. This is particularly nice served with artichokes.

TOMATO VINAIGRETTE
makes enough to dress a salad for 8
This oil-free vinaigrette is particularly good on a green salad.

What you need
160 ml (5 1/2 fl oz) tomato juice
3 tsp balsamic vinegar
1 tbsp wine vinegar
2 garlic cloves, crushed
1 tsp onion salt
10 leaves of fresh basil or tarragon
10 leaves of broad-leaved parsley
1 tbsp tamari (or more to taste)
freshly ground black pepper

Here's how
Blend all the ingredients in a food processor, then season to taste.

GINGER DRESSING
makes enough to dress a salad for 4
Another dip-dressing, this one has a fine hot flavour perfect for a green salad.

What you need
100 g (4 oz) of tofu
juice of 1 lemon
zest of 1 lemon, finely shredded
1 tsp honey
1 tsp grated ginger root
1 garlic clove, crushed
1 tbsp red wine
1 tsp vegetable bouillon powder

Here's how
Blend all the ingredients well in a food processor. Alter the quantity of red wine to adjust the thickness.

FRENCH DRESSINGS
These dressings are especially good for leafy salads such as lettuce and spinach. With the right seasonings such as a tasty mustard and various herbs, they can be very flavourful and not at all the 'plain oil and vinegar dressing' most people know.

BASIC FRENCH DRESSING
makes enough to dress a salad for 8

What you need
175 ml (6 fl oz) tomato juice
4 tbsp lemon juice or cider vinegar
1 tsp wholegrain mustard or mustard powder

a little vegetable bouillon powder or tamari
1 garlic clove, crushed or a dried tarragon leaf
freshly ground black pepper

Here's how
Combine the ingredients in a processor or simply place in a screw-top jar and shake well to mix. Sometimes I like to thin this dressing and make it a little lighter by adding a couple of tablespoons of water.

SPICY FRENCH DRESSING
makes 125 ml (4 fl oz)
This is a pleasant light dressing that seems to complement almost any salad.

What you need
juice of 2 lemons
2 ripe tomatoes
1 garlic clove
12 chives, finely chopped
1 tsp powdered kelp (optional)
6 tbsp walnut oil or extra-virgin olive oil
1 tbsp tamari
1/4 tsp cayenne
1 tbsp Dijon mustard
1 tsp vegetable bouillon powder

Here's how
Blend together the salad dressing by placing all of the ingredients in a food processor and mixing thoroughly. Pour the dressing over the salad, mix well and serve immediately. This dressing may be refrigerated and kept for up to four days.

CITRUS DRESSING
makes enough to dress a salad for 4

What you need
75 g (3 oz) seasoned tofu
juice of 1/2 lemon
juice of 1 orange
1 tbsp vinegar
pinch of nutmeg
1 tsp chervil
1 tsp honey
Maldon sea salt and freshly ground pepper
zest of 1/2 lemon, shredded fine
zest of 1/2 orange, shredded fine

Here's how
Blend together all ingredients except the citrus zests until smooth. Then add the zests and mix by hand.

RESOURCES

Leslie Kenton lectures and teaches workshops throughout the world on health, creativity and spirituality. Her series of Journey to Freedom Workshops on spirituality provide tools, techniques and inspiration needed to access authentic personal power and freedom. They are based on leading-edge consciousness research, emerging paradigm science, world mythology and shamanism.

If you wish to have more information about these workshops, or know about Leslie's personal appearances, forthcoming books, videos, workshops and projects, please visit her website for worldwide information: www.qed-productions/lesliekenton.htm, or write to her, enclosing a stamped, self-addressed, A4 envelope to: Leslie Kenton, Blue Dolphins, Manorbier, Pembrokeshire SA70 7SW. Telephone (44) 183 487 1447, Fax (44) 183 487 1614, e-mail: lesliekenton.office@virgin.net.

Leslie's audio tape set *10 Steps to a New You* can be ordered from **QED Recording Services Ltd,** Lancaster Road, New Barnet, Hertfordshire, EN4 8AS. Telephone (44) 181 441 7722, Fax (44) 181 441 077, e-mail: qed@globalnet.co.uk.

Journey to Freedom is now also available on audio tape from bookshops or direct from **Thorsons'** 24-hour telephone ordering service: (44) 181 307 4052 or (44) 141 306 3349.

BONSOY SOYA MILK: the very best soya milk in the world, unusual in that it is not packed in aluminium. It can be purchased from **Freshlands,** 196 Old Street, London, EC1V 9FR. Tel: 020 7250 1708. Or from Wild Oats, 210 Westbourne Grove, London, W11 2RH. Tel: 020 7229 1063.

GINSENG: My favourite ginseng comes in the form of a granulated Jinlin Ginseng Tea, which comes in sachets. Jinlin also do Panax ginseng dried slices, ampoules and whole root, available from health food stores. They also do ginseng tea in bags. If you have difficulty finding it, contact **Alice Chiu,** Man Shuen Hong (London) Ltd, 4 Tring Close, Barkingside, Essex, IG2 7LQ. Telephone: 020 8550 9900, fax: 020 8554 3883.

GREEN SUPPLEMENTS: Pure Synergy and other good green products are available mail order from **Xynergy Health Products,** Elsted, Midhurst, West Sussex GU29 0JT. Telephone: 01730 813642, fax: 01730 815109, website: www.xynergy.co.uk. Pure Synergy is simply the best nutritional supplement I have ever seen, a mix of 62 organically grown superfoods working together synergistically to support life-energy in its purest form.
Chlorella is available in vegi-capsule form from **Solgar Vitamin & Herb,** who also do an excellent green supplement 'Earth Source Green & More' in powder or tablet form. For your local stockist contact: **Solgar Vitamin & Herb,** Aldbury, Tring, Herts, HP23 5PT. Telephone: 01442 890355, fax: 01442 890366, website: www.solgar.com.

HERB TEAS: Some of my favourite blends include Cinnamon Rose, Orange Zinger and Emperor's Choice by Celestial Seasonings; Warm & Spicy by Symmingtons, and Creamy Carob French Vanilla. Yogi Tea by Golden Temple Products is a strong spicy blend, perfect as a coffee replacement. **GREEN TEA** is available from health food stores and Oriental supermarkets.

HONEY: The New Zealand Natural Food Company have a fine range of honey, including organic honey, in particular manuka honey, known for its anti-bacterial effects. **The New Zealand Natural Food Company Ltd,** Unit 3, 55-57 Park Royal Road, London, NW10 7LP. Telephone: 020 8961 4410, fax 020 8961 9420.
Evernat do a good organic honey from Argentina, available from **Planet Organic and good health food stores.** For stockists call 01932 354 211.
The Garvin Honey Company has a good selection of set and clear honeys from all over the world. These can be ordered from **The Garvin Honey Company Ltd,** Garvin House, 158 Twickenham Road, Isleworth, Middlesex, TW7 7LD. Telephone: 020 8560 7171.

JUICERS: Moulinex do a good inexpensive centrifugal juicer.
The Champion maticating juicer: veteran juicers wax lyrical about the virtues of the Champion, an indestructible American juicer that some people claim makes better juice than any centrifugal extractor can. The Champion is basically a rotating cutter on a shaft, which expels dry pulp from its shout at one end as the juice is drained through a nozzle underneath.
The Vita-Mix Total Nutrition Centre: Basically a turbo-charged, super-efficient blender with indestructible stainless steel blades and an extremely powerful motor, the TNC is dynamite! It's the only machine

that is properly able to make the fibre-rich juices - the kind of molecular, or total, juicing, discussed in Chapter Nine. It is also effective for making cereal grass juices (which must be strained before use). The TNC can also be used to make soups and ice cream. These American machines are expensive, but owning one could change your life. Contact **Country Life Natural Food Shop** Ltd, 3-4 Warwick Street, London W1R 5WA. Telephone: 020 7434 2922, fax: 020 7434 2838.

MALDON SALT FLAKES: Available from good health food stores and some supermarkets. This is the best tasting salt I have ever found. It is spiky and delicious to crumble.

MARIGOLD SWISS VEGETABLE BOUILLON POWDER: This instant broth made from vegetables and sea salt comes in regular, low-salt, vegan and organic varieties. It is available from health food stores, or direct from **Marigold Foods,** 102 Camley Street, London NW1 0PF. Telephone: 020 7388 4515, fax: 020 7388 4516.

ORGANIC FOODS: The Soil Association publishes a regularly updated comprehensive national directory of farm shops, box schemes, and retailers registered with the Soil Association or other recognized certification body. Called **Where to Buy Organic Foods,** it costs £5 including postage from: **The Soil Association,** Bristol House, 40-56 Victoria Street, Bristol BS1 6BY. Tel: 0117 929 0661, fax: 0117 925 2504, e-mail: info@soilassociation.org, website: www.soilassociation.org.
London Organic Food Forum: an organization at the heart of the organic

movement. The London Organic Food Forum newsletter keeps its members in touch with organic events in the capital as well as information and comment on what's going on: LOFF, The Membership Secretary, 17 Vernon Road, London N8 0QD.
Clearspring : Supply organic foods and natural remedies as well as macrobiotic foods by mail order. They have a good range of herbal teas, organic grains, whole seeds for spouting, dried fruits, pulses, nut butters, Soya and vegetable products, sea vegetables, drinks and Bioforce herb tinctures. Write to them for a catalogue: **Clearspring,** Unit 19a, Acton Park Estate, London W3 7QE. Telephone: 020 8746 0152, fax: 020 8811 8893. You can order by telephone, fax, post or shop online at www.clearspring.co.uk.
Organics Direct: Offers a nation-wide home delivery service of fresh vegetables and fruits, delicious breads, juices, sprouts, fresh soups, ready-made meals, snacks and baby foods. They also sell state-of-the-art Juicer and organic wines – all shipped to you within 24 hours.
Organics Direct, 1-7 Willow Street, London EC2A 4BH. Telephone: 020 7729 2828, fax: 020 7613 5800, website: www.organicsdirect.com. You can order online.

ORGANIC MEAT: Good quality organic beef, pork, bacon, lamb, chicken, turkey, duck and geese, a variety of types of sausage, all dairy products, vegetables and organic groceries (2000 lines), are available mail order from: **Longwood Farm Organic Meats,** Tudenham St Mary, Bury St Edmunds, Suffolk IP28 6TB. Telephone: 01638 717120, fax: 01638 717120. They also deliver other organic foods.

SEA PLANTS FOR COOKING AND SALADS: Those such as kelp, dulse, nori, kombu and wakami can be bought from Japanese grocers or macrobiotic health shops.

SHIITAKE AND MAITAKE MUSHROOMS: These are available from Japanese grocers or macrobiotic health food shops. Shi-Ta-Ke Extract in capsule form is available from **BioCare Ltd,** Lakeside, 180 Lifford Lane, Kings Norton, Birmingham, West Midlands B30 3NU. Telephone: 0121 433 3727, fax: 0121 433 3879.

UDO'S CHOICE: Organic flax, sunflower and sesame oils mechanically pressed in a low heat, light and oxygen-free environment – excellent source of essential fatty acids. Available from good health food stores.

WATER: Fresh Water 1000 Water Filter System: Getting pure water can be difficult. One in ten of us drink water that is contaminated with poisons above international standards. I have found a water purifier that I think is good, it is the Fresh Water 1000 water filter system. It removes more than 90 percent of heavy metals, pesticides and hydrocarbons such as benzene, trihalmethanes, chlorine, oestrogen and bacteria without removing essential minerals like calcium. Available from **The Fresh Water Filter Company,** Carlton House, Aylmer Road, Leytonstone, London E11 3AD. Telephone: 020 8558 7495, fax: 020 8556 9270.
Friends of the Earth have an excellent free booklet called Water Pollution. Contact: **Friends of the Earth,** 26-28 Underwood Street, London N1 7JQ. Telephone: 020 7490 1555, fax: 0207 490 0881.

FURTHER READING

Ardrey, R., *African Genesis,* Atheneum, New York, 1961.

Balch, James, M.D., and Balch, Phyllis A., *Prescription for Nutritional Healing,* Avery Publishing Group, Garden City Park, N.Y., 1990.

Ballentine, Rudolph, M.D., *Diet & Nutrition: A Holistic Approach,* Himalayan International Institute, Honesdale, P.A., 1978.

Barnard, Neal, M.D., *Food for Life: How the New Four Food Groups Can Save Your Life,* Harmony Books, New York, 1993.

Barnard, Neal, *The Power of Your Plate: A Plan for Better Living,* Book Publishing Company, Summertown, T.N., 1995.

Berger, Stuart, M.D., *Dr Berger's Immune Power Diet,* Signet/New American Library, New York, 1985.

Berglund, B., and Bolsby Clare, *Edible Wild Plants,* Charles Scribner's Sons, New York, 1977.

Beyer, Bee, *Food Drying at Home the Natural Way,* J.P. Tarcher, Inc., Los Angeles, 1976.

Bianchini, Francesco, and Corbetta, Francesco, *Health Plants of the World,* Newsweek Books, New York, 1977.

Bianchini, Francesco, et al., *The Complete Book of Fruits and Vegetables,* Crown Publishers, New York, 1975.

Black, Helen, ed., *The Berkeley Co-op Food Book,* Bull Publishing Company, Palo Alto, C.A., 1980.

Blue Goose Buying Guide for Fresh Fruits, Vegetables, and Nuts, Blue Goose, Inc., Hagerstown, M.D.

Bolitho, Hector, *The Glorious Oyster,* Sidgwick and Jackson, London, 1960.

Born, Wina, *The Concise Atlas of Wine,* Charles Scribner's Sons, New York, 1972.

Brecher, Edward M., *Licit and Illicit Drugs,* Little, Brown and Company, Boston, 1972.

Carper, Jean, *Food: Your Miracle Medicine,* Harper Perrenial, New York, 1994.

Carper, Jean, *Stop Aging Now! The Ultimate Plan for Staying Young & Reversing the Aging Process,* Harper Collins, New York, 1995.

Cheraskin, E., Ringsdorf W.M., Jr., and Brecher Arline, Psychodietetics, *Bantam Books,* New York, 1974.

Ciba Foundation Symposium 22 (New Series), *Aromatic Amino Acids in the Brain,* Associated Scientific Publishers, Amsterdam, 1974.

Clark, Linda, *Know Your Nutrition,* Keats Publishing, New Canaan, C.T., 1981.

Coon, C. S., *The Hunting Peoples,* Little, Brown and Company, Boston, 1971.

Coyle, L. Patrick, Jr., *The World Encyclopedia of Food, Facts on File,* New York, 1982.

Davies, David, *The Centenarians of the Andes,* Anchor Press/Doubleday, Garden City, N.Y., 1975.

Davis, Myrna, *The Potato Book,* William Morrow & Co., New York, 1973.

Davison, A. N., ed. *Biochemical Correlates of Brain Structure and Function,* Academic Press, New York, 1977.

Eccles, John, *The Understanding of the Brain,* McGraw-Hill Book Company, New York, 1973.

Encyclopedia of Organic Gardening, Rodale Press, Emmaus, P.A., 1976.

Erasmus, Udo, *Fats and Oils: The Complete Guide to Fats and Oils in Health and Nutrition,* Alive Publishing, Vancouver, 1986.

Evans, T., and Greene D., *The Meat Book,* Charles Scribner's Sons, New York, 1973.

Ewald, Ellen Buchman, *Recipes for a Small Planet,* Ballantine Books, New York, 1973.

Fries, James F., and Crapo, Lawrence M., *Vitality and Aging,* W.H. Freeman and Company, New York, 1981.

Froud, Nina, *The World Book of Vegetable, Rice & Pasta Dishes,* Pelharn Books Ltd., London, England, 1969.

Fryer, L., and Dickinson, A., *A Dictionary of Food Supplements,* Mason-Charter, New York, 1975.

Garrison, Robert H., Jr., and Somet, Elizabeth, *The Nutrition Desk Reference,* 3rd ed., Keats Publishing, New Canaan, C.T., 1995.

Goldbeck, Nikki and David, *American Wholefoods Cuisine,* Plume/New American Library, New York, 1983.

Goldberg, Israel, ed. *Functional Foods: Designer Foods,* Pharmafoods, Nutraceuticals, Chapman & Hall, New York, 1994.

Hagiwara, Yoshihide, M.D., *Green Barley Essence,* Keats Publishing, New Canaan, C.T., 1985.

Hallowell, Michael, *Herbal Healing: A Practical Introduction to Medicinal Herbs,* Avery Publishing Group, Garden City Park, N.Y., 1994.

Harris, B.C., *Kitchen Medicines,* Pocket Books, New York, 1970.

Harris, R. S., and Von Loldcke, H., eds. *Nutritional Evaluation of Food Processing,* Avi Publishing, Westport, Conn., 1971.

Harrison, Lewis, *Making Fats and Oils Work for You,* Avery Publishing Group, Garden City Park, N.Y., 1990.

Hausman, Patricia, and Hurley, Judith Benn, *The Healing Foods,* Rodale Press, Emmaus, P.A., 1989.

Heinerman, John, *The Healing Benefits of Garlic,* Keats Publishing, New Canaan, C.T., 1994.

Hendrickson, Robert, *The Great American Tomato Book,* Doubleday & Company, Garden City, N.Y., 1976.

Henrikson, Robert, *Earth Food Spirulina,* Ronore Enterprises, Laguna Beach, C.A., 1989.

Hill, H., *Ninety-Nine Miracle Food Products of Nature,* Castle Books, Secaucus, New Jersey, 1973.

Hoffman, David, *An Elder's Herbal: Natural Techniques for Promoting Health and Vitality,* Healing Arts Press, Rochester, V.T., 1993.

Hur, Robin, *Food Reform: Our Desperate Need,* Heidelberg Publishing, Austin, Tex., 1973.

Kadans, Joseph, *Encyclopedia of Fruits, Vegetables, Nuts and Seeds for Healthful Living,* Parker Publishing, West Nyack, N.Y., 1973.

Lang, Jennifer Harvey, ed. Larousse Gastronomique: *The New American Edition of the World's Greatest Culinary Encyclopedia, Crown Publishers,* New York, 1988.

Lappe, Francis Moore, *Diet for a Small Planet,* Tenth anniversary edition, Ballantine Books, New York, 1982.

Lehane, B., *The Power of Plants,* McGraw-Hill, Maidenhead, England, 1977.

Lin, David J., *Free Radicals and Disease Prevention: What You Must Know,* Keats Publishing, New Canaan, C.T., 1993.

Lucas, Jack, *Our Polluted Food,* Charles Knight and Company, London, 1975.

Lucra, S., *Medicinal Uses of Wine,* Wine Advisory Board of California, 1972.

Mallard, Gwen, *Soya Bean Magic: Delicious Recipes with Soya Beans, Flour & Grits,* Hancock House Publishers, Ltd., Saanichton, British Columbia, 1976.

Messina, Mark, and Messina, Virginia, *The Simple Soybean and Your Health,* Avery Publishing Group, Garden City Park, N.Y., 1994.

Mowrey, Daniel B., *The Scientific Validation of Herbal Medicine,* Cormorant Books, 1986.

Rath, Matthias, M.D., *Eradicating Heart Disease, Health Now,* San Francisco, 1993.

Rodale's Basic Natural Foods Cookbook, Rodale Press, Emmaus, P.A., 1984.

Rosenthal, Sylvia, *Fresh Food,* E. P. Dutton, New York, 1978.

Salaman, Maureen, *Foods That Heal,* M.K.S., Menlo Park, C.A., 1989.

Schulick, Paul, *Common Spice or Wonder Drug?,* Herbal Free Press, Brauleboro, V.T., 1994.

Seibold, Ronald, *Cereal Grass: What's in It for You!,* Wilderness Community Education Foundation, Lawrence, K.S., 1990.

Seibold, Ronald, ed. *Cereal Grass: Nature's Greatest Health Gift,* Keats Publishing, New Canaan, C.T., 1991.

Sharma, Hari, M.D., *Freedom from Disease: How to Control Free Radicals,* Veda Publishing, Toron to, 1993.

Shurtleff, William, and Aoyagi, Akiko, *Book of Miso,* Ballantine Books, New York, 1982.

Simon, Andre L., *A Concise Encyclopedia of Gastronomy,* Overlook Press, Woodstock, N.Y., 1981.

Simon, Andre L., and Howe, Robin, *Dictionary of Gastronomy,* Overlook Press, Woodstock, N.Y., 1978.

Tyler, Varro E., *Herbs of Choice: The Therapeutics use of Phytochemicals,* Pharmaceutical Products Press, New York, 1994.

Tyler, Varro E., *The Honest Herbal: A Sensible Guide to the Use of Herbs and Related Remedies,* Pharmaceutical Products Press, New York, 1993.

Walcher, D. N., Kretchmer, N., and Barnett, H. L., *Food, Man and Society,* Plenum Press, New York, 1976.

Ward, Artemus, *Encyclopedia of Food,* Peter Smith, New York, 1941.

Weiss, Theodore J., Ph.D., *Food Oils and Their Uses, 2d ed.,* AVI Publishing Co., Westport, C.T., 1982.

Wheelwright, E. G., *Medicinal Plants and Their History,* Dover Publications, New York, 1974.

Whitaker, Julian, M.D., Dr. *Whitaker's Guide to Natural Healing,* Prima Publishing, Rocklin, C.A., 1995.

Whole Foods Magazine, *Natural Foods Guide, And/Or Press, Berkeley,* C.A., 1979.

Wilson, C. O., and Grisvold, O., *Texbook of Organic Medical and Pharmaceutical Chemistry,* J. B. Lippincott, Philadelphia, 1956.

Wood, Rebecca, *The Whole Foods Encyclopedia: A Shopper's Guide,* Prentice Hall, New York, 1988.

Wright, Jonathan, M.D., *Dr. Wright's Guide to Healing with Nutrition,* Keats Publishing, New Canaan, C.T.,1990.

Yu Lu, *The Classic of Tea,* Little, Brown and Company, Boston, 1974.

THE INDEX

Page numbers in **bold** represent photographs

ACKNOWLEDGMENTS

From beginning to end, this book has been sheer pleasure for me to write and photograph. Partly this may be because little is more wonderful to work with and play with than organically grown fresh fruits and vegetables, seafood, game, pulses and grains. My pleasure in sharing my recipes with you has been much increased by my working with an enormously talented and supportive group of people without whom the book simply would never have happened.

At the top of the list are my editor Denise Bates and publisher Amelia Thorpe, whose idea the book was in the first place. And most of all to Gail Rebuck, whose love of my photographs pulled out all the stops to find the best way to display them and the best people to help me get the visual aspect of the book right.

Amanda Cooper Davies, one of the most talented food stylists, worked with me on all the photographs and taught me – a budding food photographer – how to attempt the impossible in a way that was more fun than I would ever imagine it could be.

Shirley Bradstock bought the food and prepared and cooked all these wonderful dishes. She is not only a skilled cook but a woman of enormous energy and passion which she brings to everything we do together.

Judith Stoothoff painstakingly typed all of my words and edited them again and again on computer – cheerfully and professionally, while her husband Bob worked out how to communicate between Judith's Mac and my PC – not an easy marriage to handle in anybody's book.

My thanks go to David Eldridge, the book's designer, for his passion and his willingness to work with the photos and the words until he got it right. This was no mean task when so many of us were asking him to do the impossible day after day.

Meanwhile, Emma Callery has once again faced the challenge of my impossible spelling and off-the-wall measurements to do the impossible and make of my rough words the equivalent of a silk purse from a sow's ear.

And what of the others – stretching back sometimes thirty years – doctors and biochemists who have taught me and continue to teach me about the nutritional value of the foods used in these recipes? To list them all would fill a book in itself. Suffice it to say that I am enormously grateful to you all for your support and encouragement, your wisdom and your skills. Thank you.

Leslie Kenton
London 2001